Essentials of Health Economics

Diane M. Dewar, PhD

Associate Professor
Department of Economics and
Department of Health Policy, Management and Behavior
School of Public Health
University at Albany—State University of New York
Albany, New York

JONES AND BARTLETT PUBLISHERS
Sudbury, Massachusetts
BOSTON   TORONTO   LONDON   SINGAPORE

World Headquarters
Jones and Bartlett Publishers
40 Tall Pine Drive
Sudbury, MA 01776
978-443-5000
info@jbpub.com
www.jbpub.com

Jones and Bartlett Publishers
Canada
6339 Ormindale Way
Mississauga, Ontario L5V 1J2
Canada

Jones and Bartlett Publishers
International
Barb House, Barb Mews
London W6 7PA
United Kingdom

Jones and Bartlett's books and products are available through most bookstores and online booksellers. To contact Jones and Bartlett Publishers directly, call 800-832-0034, fax 978-443-8000, or visit our website, www.jbpub.com.

Substantial discounts on bulk quantities of Jones and Bartlett's publications are available to corporations, professional associations, and other qualified organizations. For details and specific discount information, contact the special sales department at Jones and Bartlett via the above contact information or send an email to specialsales@jbpub.com.

This publication is designed to provide accurate and authoritative information in regard to the Subject Matter covered. It is sold with the understanding that the publisher is not engaged in rendering legal, accounting, or other professional service. If legal advice or other expert assistance is required, the service of a competent professional person should be sought.

Production Credits
Publisher: Michael Brown
Associate Editor: Katey Birtcher
Editorial Assistant: Catie Heverling
Senior Production Editor: Tracey Chapman
Senior Marketing Manager: Sophie Fleck
Manufacturing and Inventory Control Supervisor: Amy Bacus
Composition: Auburn Associates, Inc.
Cover Design: Kristin E. Parker
Cover Image: Clockwise from top left: © Andreea Ardelean/Dreamstime.com; © Rorem/Dreamstime.com; © Dimitry Romanchuck/Dreamstime.com; © Haak 78/Dreamstime.com
Printing and Binding: Malloy, Inc.
Cover Printing: John Pow Company

Library of Congress Cataloging-in-Publication Data
Dewar, Diane M.
  Essentials of health economics / Diane M. Dewar.
    p. ; cm. — (Essential public health series)
  Includes bibliographical references and index.
  ISBN-13: 978-0-7637-3797-9 (pbk.)
  ISBN-10: 0-7637-3797-6 (pbk.)
 1. Medical economics—United States. I. Title. II. Series: Essential public health.
  [DNLM: 1. Economics, Medical—United States. 2. Delivery of Health Care—economics—United States. 3. Insurance, Health—economics—United States. W 74 AA1 D515e 2010]
  RA410.53.D49 2010
  338.4′73621—dc22
                                                                                          2009000083

6048
Printed in the United States of America
13 12 11 10 09   10 9 8 7 6 5 4 3 2 1

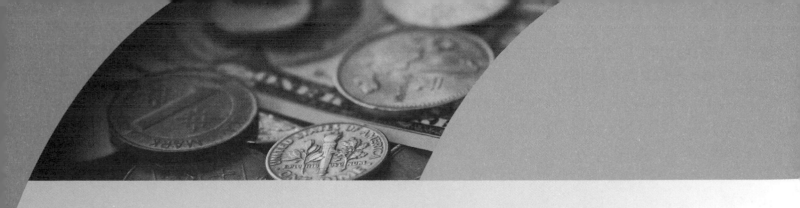

Dedication

To the two most influential women in my life:
The mother who raised me and the sister who inspired me.
Elizabeth W. Dewar
Christina E. Clothier

Acknowledgments

As the sole author of this book, I take full responsibility for its contents. However, a project of this size could not be completed by a single person. I owe a great deal to my colleagues in the Writer's Club at the School of Public Health at the University at Albany, for their patience and constructive criticisms of the earlier drafts of this work. Also, the support of the other authors in the *Essential Public Health Series*, as well as the Series Editor, Richard Riegelman of The George Washington University, who gave me the inspiration to complete the project. I am additionally appreciative of the anonymous reviewers' comments. They were all invaluable in the book's development.

I am also grateful to the numerous graduate and undergraduate students at the University at Albany, who used sections of this book in manuscript form. Their willingness to use and help revise a work in progress will benefit countless other students who work with this book in the future.

Finally, I could have never completed the book without the support and understanding of my family. Thank you all for your love and patience, and Jack, I look forward to having you in class when you get older.

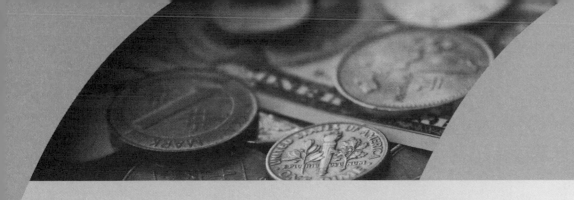

Contents

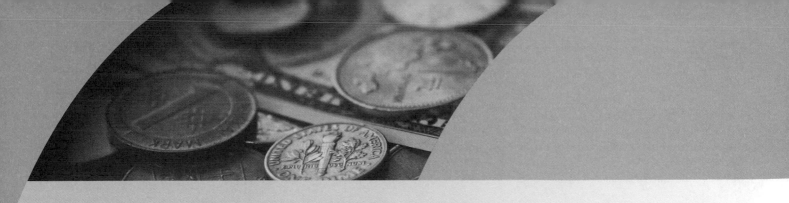

The Essential Public Health Series

*Log on to **www.essentialpublichealth.com** for the most current information on availability.*

CURRENT AND FORTHCOMING TITLES IN THE *ESSENTIAL PUBLIC HEALTH SERIES*:

ABOUT THE EDITOR:

Richard K. Riegelman, MD, MPH, PhD, is Professor of Epidemiology Biostatistics, Medicine, and Health Policy, and Founding Dean of The George Washington University School of Public Health and Health Services in Washington,

DC. He has taken a lead role in developing the Educated Citizen and Public Health initiative which has brought together arts and sciences and public health education associations to implement the Institute of Medicine of the National Academies recommendation that ". . .all undergraduates should have access to education in public health." Dr. Riegelman also led the development of George Washington's undergraduate major and minor and currently teaches "Public Health 101" and "Epidemiology 101" to undergraduates.

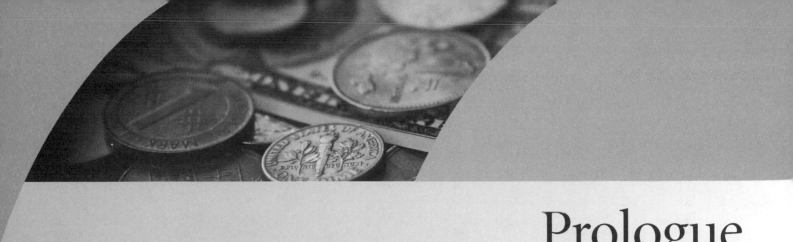

Prologue

Money talks and we need to listen if we are going to improve our health system. To understand what is being said, students in public health, health administration, clinical health professions, as well as undergraduates trying to understand these fields, need to appreciate the basic principles of economics and their applications.

Essentials of Health Economics provides a step-by-step approach to appreciating the key principles and applications of economics. This book introduces you to the principles of economics as they apply to health systems. It then applies these principles to current issues of health care and public health. You come away with the tools and concepts you need to understand the debates about the future of our health system.

Dr. Dewar's style is approachable and intuitive. It does not require complicated mathematical formulae and emphasizes common sense explanations. It does not require previous courses in economics or mathematics. It does require an interest in understanding how the world really works and how we can use principles of economics to improve our health system. You will take away an enduring understanding that will serve you well whether you become a public health professional, a healthcare administrator, a clinician, or an educated and interested citizen.

I am pleased that *Essentials of Health Economics* has joined our *Essential Public Health* book series. It complements our growing list of books designed to cover the spectrum of introductory courses to help students understand and hopefully improve our health system.

Health economics is not the dismal science that once described economics. It is an everyday tool that will help you find your way through the maze of public health and healthcare issues. Give it a try—it's well worth your time.

Richard Riegelman, MD, MPH, PhD
Series Editor

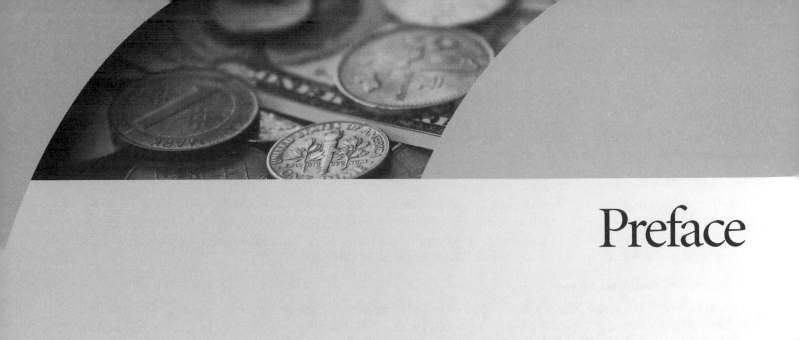

Preface

This book addresses the important economic and public health policy issues that serve as the background for the healthcare debate concerning access to a healthcare system dominated by managed care.

The primary goals of this book are to enable undergraduate students to:

1. recognize the relevance of economics to health care and to apply economic reasoning to better understand health care and health-related issues
2. understand the mechanisms of healthcare delivery in the United States and other countries within broad social and economic contexts
3. explore the changing nature of health care, health-related technology, and workforce planning, and their implications for medical practice and public health policy
4. analyze public health policy issues in the healthcare sector from an economic perspective

To accomplish these goals, the book's 17 chapters are organized into the following six parts:

What Is Health Economics?

The text begins with a basic overview of the United States healthcare system emphasizing economic issues that affect healthcare delivery and finance. Chapter 1 examines the main system level issues and the organization of the system. Chapter 2 demonstrates the usefulness of economics in understanding healthcare issues, including matters of life and death.

Demand

Part II examines the demand side of the healthcare economy. Chapters 3 and 4 present the factors that influence the demands for health and health care. It explores the observed patterns in the quality and price of health care. Chapter 5 discusses the market for health insurance, including the private and social insurance models.

Supply

Part III discusses various aspects of the supply side of the healthcare economy. Chapter 6 describes the factors that influence the production, costs, and supply of services. Chapter 7 presents the market for healthcare personnel, namely physicians and nurses, as well as the factors that influence the behavior of healthcare personnel. Chapter 8 explores the role of technological innovation and diffusion in the healthcare sector, and the reasons why technology is a major factor in the rising costs of health care.

Healthcare Markets

Part IV examines the competitive market in Chapter 9, as well as the role of government interventions to correct for failures in the competitive market in Chapter 10.

Issues in Health Economics

Part V discusses three aspects of the healthcare system: the role of socioeconomic factors in the demands on the healthcare system (Chapter 11), the significant impact of the hospital sector on the health economy (Chapter 12), and the current status of the biopharmaceutical industry (Chapter 13). All of these issues have a large impact on the actual growth of the health economy, as well as the perceptions of what is included in the growth of this sector.

Evaluating the Healthcare System

This final part explores analytical methods of evaluation, as well as the role of healthcare reform in the attempt to contain costs in the healthcare economy. Chapter 14 presents the models for economic evaluation, and Chapter 15 compares the healthcare systems of the United States, Canada, Germany, the United Kingdom, as well as Singapore via a case study. Chapter 16 discusses healthcare reform motivations and initiatives at the state and national levels. Chapter 17 summarizes the major lessons learned from the economic approach to public health policy and makes recommendations for reform of the healthcare system.

Pedagogical Features and Level

There is tremendous excitement in the healthcare field, such as the transformation of organizational arrangements, medical technology advances, the development of new healthcare financing mechanisms, and the evaluation of the healthcare system policies that lend themselves to economic analysis. This book takes a timely approach to the study of the public healthcare system through the lens of economics. Students and faculty will be able to grasp the importance and relevance of health economics, as well as how it relates to more general analysis of health policy issues, from numerous examples throughout the text. This book has widespread appeal among students of public health and health administration, since it conveys the essence of the economic issues at hand while avoiding complicated methodological issues that would interest only students of economics.

It is written with the nonspecialist in mind, while focusing on descriptive, explanatory, and evaluative economics in a systematic way. This book is accessible to undergraduates who do not have much prior knowledge of health economics or mathematics. It will be a useful introductory health economics text that does not require any other economics prerequisites. The text would be appropriate for students in the following areas: in a school of public health, as an introductory course in health economics in an economics department, in a medical, nursing, or pharmacy school, or in a health administration program.

Diane M. Dewar, PhD

About the Author

Diane M. Dewar, PhD, is an associate professor in the Department of Health Policy, Management, and Behavior of the School of Public Health, and the Department of Economics at the University at Albany, State University of New York. She has over 15 years of teaching experience which includes graduate courses in health economics, health policy and economic evaluation methods, as well as undergraduate courses in microeconomics, macroeconomics, econometrics, health economics, comparative health policy, introductory sociology, and introductory psychology.

Professor Dewar received her PhD in economics from the University at Albany, with concentrations in health economics and econometrics. She is a recipient of the William Waters Research Award from the Association of Social Economists, received an honorable mention for the Aetna Susan B. Anthony Award for Research on Older Women from the Gerontological Section of the American Public Health Association, and is a member of the Public Health Honor Society, Delta Omega, Alpha Gamma Chapter. She has been a principal investigator or co-investigator on grants from the Agency for Healthcare Research and Quality, the Robert Wood Johnson Foundation, the Kaiser Family Foundation, and the Centers for Disease Control and Prevention. She is the past Chair of the National Fellowship Panel of the American Association of University Women, has served on Agency for Healthcare Research and Quality grant review study groups, and serves on the Health Economics Committee of the Medical Care Section of the American Public Health Association.

Professor Dewar has provided extensive service to the University community. She served on numerous departmental, school, and university committees, such as belonging to the departmental and university curriculum committees, chairing the School of Public Health Council, chairing the University Council on Promotion and Continuing Appointments, serving as a University Senate Chair, chairing the School of Public Health Student Affairs Committee, and working on an undergraduate minor in public health policy and economics. For these efforts, she is the recipient of the University at Albany Excellence in Academic Service Award, as well as the State University of New York Chancellor's Award for Academic Excellence.

Professor Dewar is also an ad hoc reviewer for journals that include: *Medical Care, Annals of Internal Medicine, CHEST,* and *Critical Care Medicine.* She has authored or co-authored many articles and book chapters regarding technology assessments for those with respiratory diseases, health insurance access, and the social economy of medical care. She is also a two-time recipient of letters of commendation from the *Annals of Internal Medicine* and *CHEST* for her service as a referee for those journals.

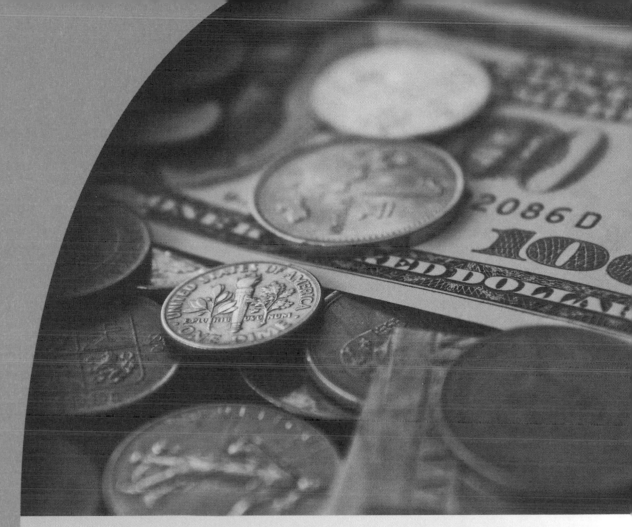

PART I

WHAT IS HEALTH ECONOMICS?

U.S. Healthcare System Issues

CHARACTERISTICS OF THE U.S. HEALTHCARE SYSTEM

Drawing heavily from Shi and Singh (2005), the U.S. healthcare system is influenced by the political climate, economic development, technological innovation and diffusion, social values, the physical environment, and demographic trends. The U.S. system is different from other countries' systems on eight dimensions:

1. There is no central governing agency and little coordination.
2. The delivery system is technology driven and focused on acute care.
3. The system is high cost, but only yields average health outcomes.
4. Health care is delivered under imperfect market conditions.
5. The private sector is the dominant market.
6. Market goals and social justice are in conflict.
7. There are multiple organizational forms and players.
8. There is a quest for integration and accountability.

All of these characteristics lead, in concert, to a dysfunctional healthcare system. The issues below describe the main areas for improvement in the system.

SYSTEM IN NEED OF REFORM

The concern over the future of health care revolves around three broad issues: cost, quality, and access. As private health insurance declines and the number of uninsured people steadily rise, emerging public consensus is that the system is in need of reform. Gaps in coverage, combined with the upward trend in medical care spending over the past several decades, add to the commonly-held belief that the U.S. healthcare system is in crisis. Many are concerned over access to care for the uninsured and the prospects for continued access for those currently with insurance.

Recent polls indicate that most insured Americans are satisfied with the quality of their own health insurance; In fact, over 80 percent of Americans said that the health care that they or their family received during the past year was good to excellent. Access, on the other hand, is a real concern. About one-half are concerned that if they become seriously ill, they will not be able to afford the health care they need (Donelan et al., 1999).

Those without insurance coverage who lack the resources to pay out of pocket must rely on public assistance and private charity for the care that they receive. Even those with health insurance lack the assurance of continued coverage. It is not contradictory for a survey respondent to be satisfied with the coverage that they receive, but to be dissatisfied with the system as a whole. Because most workers receive their health insurance as an employee benefit, losing a job means losing access to health care, which adds to the insecurity of the middle class in an era of slow job growth, corporate downsizing, and intense international competition for jobs.

Experts themselves are quite divided on the cause of the healthcare crisis. Some consider the unrestrained use of technology as the problem. Others believe that the culprits are the increased use of health insurance and tax subsidies encouraging individuals to over insure (Blendon et al., 1993).

Although the uninsured have fewer services and less coordinated care, they do have access to high quality medical care through public clinics and hospital emergency rooms. Traditionally, indigent care has been found to be directly financed by taxpayers and private charities and indirectly by shifting costs to those with insurance coverage. In fact, over one-half of the uninsured state that they have no trouble getting the health care that they need for free (Donelan et al., 1999).

Health Care

Health care is an output in which certain inputs or factors of production are combined in varying quantities—usually under a physician's supervision. The inputs include provider services, medical equipment, and pharmaceuticals. Much of the difficulty in measuring the healthcare process stems from the issue of quality and intensity. If we measure physician care by the number of patient visits to a physician's office, two brief visits count as two visits, while one brief visit and one intense visit (e.g., including diagnostic testing and treatment) also count as two visits even though more health care was provided.

In the United States, spending passed the $1 trillion mark in 1997 and currently accounts for just over 15 percent of the U.S. Gross Domestic Product (GDP). Forecasts by the Office of the Actuary at the Centers for Medicare and Medicaid Services (2005) suggest that spending on health care will account for $3.6 trillion—nearly one-fifth of all U.S. economic activity—by 2014. Researchers from the National Bureau of Economic Research suggest that it is entirely possible that health care spending will reach 33 percent of GDP by the middle of the 21st century (Hall and Jones, 2004).

Quality

Quality is a broad term and is elusive in its meaning (Donabedian, 1988). For example, organizations can have very different structural characteristics. They can differ in the training of their staff or their equipment. They can also differ in their processes of delivering health care, such as the amount of personal attention paid to providing care to individuals. The third set of characteristics includes outcomes, such as the accu-

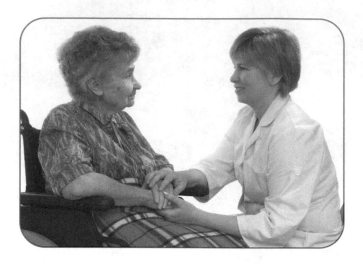

racy of the diagnoses and the techniques in treating the person and its impact on health status. This includes facility mortality and morbidity rates, and rates of adverse events such as infections or other complication rates due to a particular episode of care received. All of these aspects are considered aspects of quality. The challenge, then, is in choosing the particular aspect of quality to measure. For this reason, "visits" should only be cautiously used as a measure of physician care. Despite this challenge, physician visits are used as a measure of medical care and hospital admissions are used as a measure of output of hospital services—mostly due to their being readily available.

Outputs

Output measurements are usually conducted to make comparisons, either against other output measures or against some standard measure. There are two types of output comparisons: time series and cross-sectional comparisons. A time series comparison measures the output of the same commodity at different times, and cross-sectional comparisons measure many different outputs (e.g., health care provided by different providers or in different sociodemographic groups) during the same time period.

Health care output can be measured at three sources:

1. The providers can determine the amount of health care that they produce.
2. The payers can determine the amount of healthcare expenditures.
3. The consumers can determine the amount of health care consumed and the quality of the care consumed.

With perfect measurement, data from all three sources would be consistent. However, due to different data sources and difficulty in measuring health care, substantial variation among the sources arises.

An alternative way to measuring physician output is to focus on procedures or services. Procedures, such as tonsillectomies, can be measured in a number of ways. For example, complexity and time of performing the procedure can be used and weights can be developed for each procedure based on these dimensions (Hsiao and Stason, 1979; Hsiao et al., 1992). This approach can better capture physician tasks.

Health Insurance

Another type of healthcare sector output is risk shifting through the purchase of health insurance. Risk and uncertainty come into play in that illnesses are often unexpected and are often accompanied by monetary losses. These losses are comprised of income losses, healthcare expenses, and other expenses. Individuals are at risk of losing some of their wealth, which means that the existence of the loss and its amount are uncertain. This risk creates concern on the part of consumers and they are usually willing to pay something to avoid the risk.

One way of dealing with the risk is to shift it to another party. Insurers are organizations that specialize in accepting risk. When an insurer accepts a large amount of risk, the average loss to the insurer becomes predictable. Of course, there are costs of operating such a **risk-sharing** organization. These include the administrative expenses associated with determining probabilities, setting prices, selling policies, and adjudicating claims. The owners also expect a return on their investment, or a profit. These expenses and profits are included in the premium. The main point is that health insurance is its own output in addition to health care. An individual can obtain health care without shifting risk onto the insurer by paying for the services out of pocket when the product or service is received. Such a person is still faced with the risk of incurring losses, but nothing is done to shift the risk to a third party. Here, the action of shifting the risk reduces the loss should an illness occur.

Health insurance theoretically can cover all of a person's healthcare expenses. However, because full health insurance (i.e., the coverage for all healthcare expenses) has become costly, individuals and insurers engage in cost sharing. These provisions allow the insurers to limit expected payouts and charge the insured lower premium rates.

Cost sharing can be done in a number of ways. The individual may be required to pay a deductible of $50 before the payment from the insurer begins. The insurer can also limit the lifetime or yearly payments it will make. For example, it may cover the first $100,000 in expenses per year, but after that point, the individual will bear the full risk of the expenses. Catastrophic insurance can be purchased in order to cover these extreme expenses. Another form of cost sharing is the **coinsurance** borne by the individual for each service. The more the individual bears the risk of the healthcare services received, the larger the coinsurance rate.

The amount and type of insurance coverage is tied to the healthcare market. Although health insurance and health care should be thought of as distinct outputs in the health economy, they affect one another. In the case of insurance, distribution issues are a cause for concern. Many employed people have no insurance and the percentage of uninsured has grown to over 14 percent. Also, the mere fact of having insurance does not guarantee that one has access to health care. Because of cost-sharing arrangements, many people covered by insurance still face substantial medical risks should they become ill.

Finally, if the cost shift was complete and there was a complete absence of cost sharing on the part of the individual, there could be market problems as well. A totally riskless insurance policy may be very expensive, because individuals are more prone to demand care when it has a $0 price (as under full insurance coverage). Because the costs of care must be fully covered by the insurer, the premiums increase to cover the costs of health care received.

Health Status

The concept of health status seems familiar to us in the sense that we can recognize a healthy glow or a well-developed physique. However, more precise measures are harder to obtain. We have not defined health precisely. Lacking a precise definition, individuals can have different opinions as to whether one person is healthier than another. An essential task of the scientific method is to obtain widespread agreement about the status of health. A definition is useful if it pinpoints the characteristics of the status we are trying to describe and eventually measure. As an effort to give some framework for the concept, the World Health Organization has defined health as "a complete state of physical, mental and social well-being, and not merely the absence of illness or disease" (Jacobs and Rapoport, 2002). This is a very broad definition and the characteristics of health suggested by it are not easy to pinpoint and measure. The definition provides three components of health to consider—a person can be physically healthy, but still lacking on the other components.

Individual Health

For many years, health was identified by the presence of disease (i.e., morbidity) or by death (i.e., mortality). Individual measures, such as the diagnosis rates for certain conditions or rates of hospitalization, were used as indicators for morbidity. Mortality was usually adjusted for age and gender. More recently, mortality has been addressed as premature mortality with the difference between expected age of death and the actual age of death being forwarded as a measure of life-years lost prematurely. Therefore, if the expected age for a male aged 30 is 75 years, the death of a 30 year old man results in a 45 year loss of life.

In recent years, the concept of health has been taking a more positive focus. Measurements of health have focused on the characteristics that we would expect in a healthy person. These characteristics include the physical functioning of a person, the ability to perform certain tasks, and the emotional and social role functioning of the individual. Because these characteristics are not distinct from each other, there has been some disagreement and challenges in developing a composite measure of health status. Some researchers have focused on physical role functioning (Boyle and Torrance, 1984), while others on the mixture of social, physical, and emotional role functioning (Breslow, 1972).

Population Health

One of the most popular population health measures is mortality rates. Mortality rates are standardized by age and/or gender and can be expressed for the entire population or for subgroups based on racial, ethnic, or geographic qualities. In all cases, death rates are falling, but the death rate for blacks is substantially above that for whites.

Increasingly, analysts have been focusing on survival time as an indicator of health status. The measure of premature deaths is considered to be one of the best population-based indicators of health. Here the analysis selected a target age below which most individuals are expected to live, and deaths that occur earlier than the target age are considered to be premature.

SUMMARY

Economists seldom hesitate in applying economic tools in a variety of circumstances to evaluate individual choice behavior. However, few economists believe the economic analysis provides all of the answers. As you progress through the chapters in this text, it will become obvious that the healthcare marketplace has many failures, making it impossible to use the strict neoclassical approach in analyzing healthcare issues. The

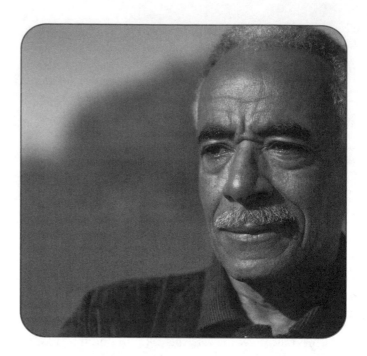

goal of this book is to show that economics can provide insights into the study of human behavior that few other disciplines offer. Specifically, human behavior is responsive to incentive and constraints. People spending others' money show little concern over how it is spent, but those spending their own money spend it more wisely.

As concerns rise over escalating costs, and the growing dysfunctionality of the healthcare system moves to the forefront, economics takes on an increasingly important role in the study of healthcare issues. As clinicians and policymakers become more versed in economic theory, the more they can shape the debate on the future of the healthcare system.

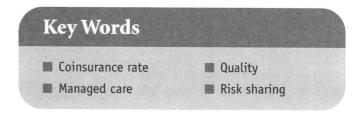

Key Words

- Coinsurance rate
- Managed care
- Quality
- Risk sharing

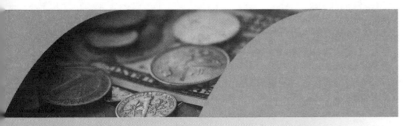

Questions

1. Distinguish between three different viewpoints of the quality of health care and provide examples of the types of care that would be considered indicators of quality for each viewpoint.

2. Specify a relationship between health care and health.

3. Why is health insurance important? Discuss what happens when people over insure or under insure.

4. What is the difference between individual and population health? What perspective would the physician use and what perspective would the policy maker use? Explain.

REFERENCES

1. Blendon, RJ, Hyams, TS, and JM Benson. (1993) Bridging the gap between expert and public views on health care reform. *Journal of the American Medical Association*, 269(19):2573–2578.

2. Boyle, MH, and GW Torrance. (1984) Developing multiattribute health indexes. *Medical Care*, 22:1045–1057.

3. Breslow, L. (1972) A quantitative approach to the World Health Organization definition of health: Physical, mental, and social well-being. *International Journal of Epidemiology*, 1:347–355.

4. Donabedian, A. (1988) The quality of care. *Journal of the American Medical Association*, 260:1743–1748.

5. Donelan, K et al. (1999) The cost of health system change: Public discontent in five nations. *Health Affairs*, 18(3):206–216.

6. Hall, JE and CI Jones. (2004) The value of life and the rise in health spending. NBER Working Paper 10737. New York: National Bureau of Economic Research. Nber.org/papers/w10737 (accessed on December 9, 2006).

7. Hsiao, WC and WB Stason. (1979) Toward developing a relative value scale for medical and surgical services. *Health Care Financing Review*, 1:23–39.

8. Hsiao, WC et al. (1992) An overview of the development and refinement of the resource-based relative value scale. *Medical Care*, 30 (Suppl.): NS1.

9. Jacobs, P and J Rapoport. (2002) *The Economics of Health and Medical Care*, 5th ed. Sudbury, MA: Jones and Bartlett Publishers.

10. Office of the Actuary at the Centers for Medicare and Medicaid Services (2005). National Health Care Expenditure Predictions 2004–2014. Current version available at cms.hhs.gov/nationalhealthexpenddata/03_natonalaccountsprojected.asp (accessed December 9, 2006).

11. Shi, L and DA Singh. (2005) *Essentials of the U.S. Health Care System*. Sudbury, MA: Jones and Bartlett Publishers.

BIO: KENNETH J. ARROW

Kenneth J. Arrow, who is primarily known for his work on general equilibrium and welfare economics, wrote what is considered by many one of the classic articles in the field of health economics. "Uncertainty and the Welfare Economics of Medical Care" (*American Economic Review*, 1963) has had as much impact on economic thinking as any single paper written in the modern era. Members of the International Health Economics Association considered his contribution so important that they named their annual award for the outstanding published paper in health economics after him.

Arrow's early work completely revolutionized the way economists think about general equilibrium and social choice. Winner of the 1972 Nobel Prize in Economics at the age of 51, he is widely considered one of the most important figures in general economic equilibrium theory and welfare theory.

Arrow's work to integrate uncertainty into economic models led to his 1963 paper on the economics of medical care. In it he was able to show that the key element in insurance markets was the difference in information between buyers and sellers of insurance. The very existence of health insurance causes individuals to spend more on medical care than they would otherwise. His emphasis on moral hazard and adverse selection served to focus in health economics on these important issues.

Arrow received his PhD in Economics from Columbia University. By the age of 32, he became a full professor at Stanford University. By the end of his first decade in academia, he was named president of the Econometric Society and winner of the John Bates Clark medal given by the American Economic Association for the most distinguished work by an economist under the age of 40.

Most of Arrow's academic career was spent at Stanford except for 11 years at Harvard University. He is currently the Joan Kenney Professor of Economics at Professor of Operations Research at Stanford University. In 1981, he was named Senior Fellow at the Hoover Institution. In addition to his many honors and affiliations, he has been president of the American Economic Association, the American Association of the Advancement of Science, and the International Economic Association.

Source: "Kenneth J. Arrow" in *Lives of the Laureates*, 3rd edition. Eds. William Breit and Roger W. Spencer (Cambridge MA: The MIT Press, 1995).

Health Economics and Policy, 2nd Edition. James W. Henderson. (Cincinnati, OH: South-western, 2002).

The Role of Economics

ECONOMICS AND POLICY

Understanding what economics can and cannot do is the first and possibly most important step in using economics as a tool of health policy. Economics can offer a framework to study the implications of individual decision making and help define the alternative mechanisms available to improve resource allocation. It cannot be used to solve all problems of healthcare access and delivery.

Sound policy making is based on sound economic principles applied in a sensitive and uniform manner. Lessons can be learned from basic economics—lessons about human behavior and the way individuals make decisions, respond to incentives, interact with each other—and about the efficient allocation of scarce resources. Economists do not have the final say about the management of the healthcare systems, but they can make important contributions to the conversation about health policy and how it relates to the healthcare system.

Even if you have had an exposure to economics, it is still important to read through this chapter. This chapter can be used to refresh your memory of the important concepts that will come into play when analyzing the medical markets and policies in these markets. This material will be useful in setting the tone for the rest of the book. The primary function of this chapter is to examine the basic principles of the market.

WHAT IS HEALTH ECONOMICS?

Health economists examine a wide range of issues from the nature and production of health to the market for health and medical care to the micro-evaluation of interventions. Grossman (1972) developed an economic framework for the study of medical care demand where medical care is simply one of many factors used to produce health. The production of health looks at the determinants of health including income, wealth, biology, public health infrastructure and interventions, and lifestyle choices. Many factors confound the ability of medical care to contribute to good health.

The principle activity of economists outside of the United States is the evaluation of medical interventions. Decision makers with limited resources find it necessary to conduct studies comparing the costs and consequences of diagnostic and treatment options to make informed decisions about efficient allocations of scarce resources. Cost-effectiveness analysis, the evaluation method of choice in medical decision making is further discussed in Chapter 14.

The primary focus of United States health economists is the **market** for health care. The demand for health care is seen as not only the desire to feel well (i.e., consumption aspects of health), but as a way to invest in human capital. Factors affecting the demand for medical care include: socioeconomic factors of the population, patient demographics, access barriers and the role of providers in determining the services to be provided. The supply of health care encompasses a broad spectrum of economics on such topics as production theory, input markets, and industrial organization. Specific issues to be examined are the cost of production, input substitution, and the nature and role of incentives. Demand and supply intersect with one another to establish market **equilibrium,** as denoted in Figure 2-1.

Markets are able to effectively allocate scarce resources where they are most productive by establishing a price for everything.

Analysis of the overall goals and objectives of the healthcare system is the subject of macroeconomic evaluations. It is here where international comparisons are made. For example, how does our system compare with other countries' systems in terms of cost, access, and quality? Health systems are constantly changing. Policy makers and planners are always looking for better ways to produce delivery and pay for a growing number of medical care services demanded by the public.

WHY HEALTH ECONOMICS IS IMPORTANT

Understanding the economics of health care is important for a number of reasons. First, health is important to us as individuals and as a society, and health care is one, though not the only, way of modifying the incidence and impact of ill health and disease. The availability of health care can determine the quality of life and the prospect for survival. Economic analysis offers a unique and systematic intellectual framework for analyzing important issues in health care and for identifying solutions to common problems. Quite literally, the economics of health care is a matter of life and death.

Secondly, the healthcare sector is very large. Health care is a major component of spending, investment, and employment in every developed country, thus, the economic performance of the healthcare system is crucially linked to the overall economic well-being of a country and its citizens (Reinhardt et al., 2002, 2004; Fuchs, 2005).

Third, decisions about how health care is funded, provided, and distributed are strongly influenced by the economic environment and economic constraints. Global, national, and local policy responses to health issues are becoming increasingly informed by economic ideas and methods of analyses. One good reason for understanding health economics is to engage in policy debates as an informed critic. For those working in health services, familiarity with the theory and methods of economic analysis is becoming essential, both to understand the context of a medical practice, and because evidence on productivity, efficiency, and value for/of money are increasingly the norm in modern healthcare systems.

Health economics is an application of economic theory, models, and empirical techniques to the analysis of decision making by individuals, healthcare providers, and governments with respect to health and health care. It is a branch of economic science—but it is not merely the application of standard economic theory to health and health care as an interesting topic. Health economics is solidly based in economic theory, but it also comprises a body of theory developed specifically to understand the behavior of patients, doctors, and hospitals, and analytical techniques developed to facilitate resource allocation decisions related to health care. Health economics has evolved into a highly specialized field, drawing on related disciplines including epidemiology, statistics, psychology, sociology, operations research, and mathematics in its approach. Alternatively, it may be regarded as an essential part of a set of analytical methods applied to health, which are usually labeled health services research.

KEY ECONOMIC CONCEPTS

These terms will serve as unifying themes throughout the text:

1. **Scarcity** addresses the problem of limited resources and the need to make choices. Rationing is unavoidable because not enough resources are available for everyone's needs. Therefore we are to choose among competing objectives—as result of scarcity.
2. **Opportunity cost** recognizes the role of alternatives. The cost of any decision or choice made is measured in terms of the value placed on the opportunity foregone.
3. **Marginal analysis** recognizes that choices are made at the margin, not on an all-or-nothing basis. In this

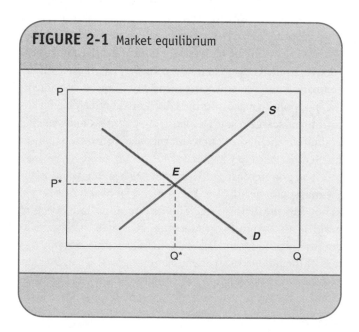

FIGURE 2-1 Market equilibrium

environment, consideration and decision making are based on incremental benefits and costs of an alternative.

5. **Self-interest** is the primary motivator of economic actors. People are motivated to pursue efficiently in the production and consumption decisions made.

6. The **Market** accomplishes its tasks through a system of prices, or the invisible hand. The invisible hand can allocate resources because everyone and everything has a price. Prices increase when more is desired, and decrease when less is desired. The price mechanism becomes a way to bring a firm's output decision into balance with consumer desires, which is the role of equilibrium.

7. **Supply and demand** serve as the foundation of economic analysis. Pricing and output decisions are based on forces underlying these two economic concepts. Rationing using prices comes about when goods and services are allocated in the market based on the consumers' willingness to pay and the suppliers' willingness to provide at a given price.

8. **Competition** forces resource owners to use their resources to promote the highest possible satisfaction of society: consumers, producers, and investors. If the resource owners do this well, they are rewarded. If they are inefficient, they are penalized. Competition takes production out of the hands of the less competitive and places into the hands of the more efficient—constantly promoting the efficient methods of production.

9. **Efficiency** measures how well resources are being used to promote social welfare. Inefficient output wastes resources while efficient use of scarce resources promotes social welfare. Social welfare is promoted through the competitive markets via the relatively independent behaviors on the part of thousands of decision makers. Consumers attempt to make themselves better off by allocating limited budgets. Producers maximize profits by using cost-minimizing methods.

10. **Market failure** arises when the free market fails to promote efficient use of resources by either producing more or less than the optimal level of output. Sources of market failure include: natural monopoly, oligopoly, externalities of production or consumption, and public goods. Other market failures can occur through violations of the competitive market, such as incomplete information and immobile resources (Santerre and Neun, 2004).

The Use of Economics in Health Care

Economics is a way to organize our thinking about problems that confront us in our daily lives. To think like an economist requires us to have a disciplined approach to a problem. Sound reasoning with systematic frameworks is essential. The value of economics stems from its usefulness in making sense out of complex economic and social issues.

Economics is one of the social sciences that attempts to explain human behavior. However, it is unique among the social sciences in that it establishes a context of scarcity and uncertainty. Specifically, economics explains how scarce resources are allocated among competing alternative uses to satisfy unlimited human wants.

The goal of economic efficiency stems from the fact that there are never enough resources to provide all the goods and services desired by society. Economists call this concept **scarcity**. Using resources in one alternative has the trade off of not being able to use the same resources in a competing activity or alternative. For example, resources applied to the health economy cannot be simultaneously applied to housing or education.

The term **opportunity costs** is defined as the potential benefit that could have been received if the resources had been used in their next best alternative. Tax dollars used to purchase medical care for the elderly cannot be used to buy education for the young. Adopting the goal of economic efficiency implies that choices should be made that maximize the total benefit from all available resources. In the health economy, this involves the evaluation of healthcare alternatives by calculating the benefits and costs of each alternative and allocating resources in a way that maximizes the net benefits to the population considered.

Economic Modeling

All scientific models start with assumptions. Economic models start by assuming that decisions are made rationally under conditions of scarcity. That is, people's actions are directed toward achieving an objective, given constraints. This assumption makes economics different from other social sciences.

In microeconomics, the assumption of rational behavior establishes a consistent framework for individual decision making. We assume that individuals must choose between competing alternatives in order to satisfy certain objectives. The problem becomes one of allocating scarce resources among these objectives. Therefore, choices must be made.

Decision makers, motivated by incentives, pursue their self-interest. Decision making is dominated by the pursuit of self-interest. Individuals use their resources to advance their own economic well-being. When confronted with alterative actions they choose the one that makes them better off. People look or the best way to achieve goals. Decision makers often practice rational ignorance, which implies that they make choices based on incomplete information. From the decision maker's perspective, the information left to be gathered costs more than its perceived worth. Scarcity is the reason that we study economics. Decisions must take into consideration foregone opportunities.

The Scientific Model:

The five basic steps in the scientific method are as follows:
1. Every analyst begins with a hypothesis based on his or her perception of how the world works. The view of the world is affected by our history, training, and cultural norms. This can introduce biases in the analyses.
2. Analysts then observe the real-world phenomena. These observations are recorded.
3. A theory is then developed to explain behavior or the phenomena or predict future behavior. These models are abstractions of reality that capture the influential features of the observed behavior.
4. The tests of hypotheses are then performed using gathered facts and data. In this step, quantitative techniques are used to promote accurate predictions.
5. Rethinking the model: If the empirical evidence is contrary to the model and its hypothesis, then the analyst may rethink the theory being tested. (Santerre and Neun, 2004).

Model Building

One of the main goals of economics is to understand, explain, and predict the actions of economic factors. In order to do this, it is necessary to simplify the behavior into its elemental parts. Simplification is accomplished through generalization and the construction of models.

A model is a way to organize knowledge and explain a particular issue in general terms. An economic model explains how a part of the economy works. Model building and theoretical developments are used interchangeably.

Microeconomic models examine the behavior of individual decision makers—individual households and firms and government agents—or specific markets. We use microeconomic models to study how patients' demands for services vary with income or insurance coverage. We can also examine the market for nurses and the effect of graduate medical education programs on the supply of physicians.

Problem Solving

Most microeconomics can be classified under the frameworks of neoclassical economics. This framework is based on optimizing behavior, which is where an economic actor is seeking

to achieve given objectives, such as profit maximization, cost minimization, or maximization of satisfaction.

Economic Optimization

When more than one alternative is available, the optimal choice produces an outcome that is most consistent with the decision maker's stated objectives. Optimization is nothing more than determining the best action given the decision maker's goals and objectives. Constrained optimization takes into account scarcity of resources. For example, how much medical care should a person consume given that his or her health insurance has changed and there are other goods and services that the person would need to purchase at a given time period?

Choices in the health economy are made at two levels: 1) individual actors must decide the best course of treatment or services to consume, and 2) policy makers must decide on the best course of action for the entire community. The health economy must consider the following questions: who to treat, when to begin treatment, where to treat, and how much treatment to offer? Of the many ways to go about finding the best alternatives, economic efficiency will be the criterion in this section.

The framework of this analysis is the neoclassical model with its assumptions of rational behavior on the part of decision makers. Firms maximize profits given technology and the costs of the resources; and consumers maximize utility or satisfaction from consuming various amounts of goods and services given limited income and the prices of goods and services considered. The labor force supplies workers in order to maximize utility from consuming goods and services and leisure time available subject to the going wage rate. This more or less independent behavior on the part of economic actors leads to equilibrium as represented in supply and demand frameworks introduced in later chapters.

Within this framework, the optimal consumption of goods and services is where the **marginal benefit** (MB) from consumption (i.e., the additional benefit received from consuming the next unit of the good or service) equals the **marginal cost** (MC) of consumption (i.e., the additional cost of consuming the next unit of a good or service).

Individuals will continue to purchase goods or services as long as $MB > MC$. Given that MB is declining and MC is rising as more of the goods or services are consumed, the two converge at some quantity. As soon as $MB = MC$, equilibrium is reached and the consumer will consume no more. This is where the additional benefit just equals the additional cost of consuming the next unit of a good or service.

From the perspective of economics, it is wasteful to consume all possible medical benefits as possible. As in Figure 2-2,

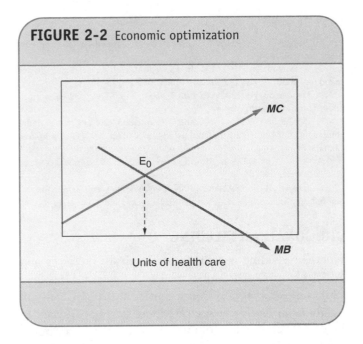

FIGURE 2-2 Economic optimization

MC

E_0

MB

Units of health care

wants involves making choices. In this world, tradeoffs are inevitable because we cannot always get what we want.

2. Medical decisions involve costs and benefits. It is essential that clinicians and policy makers have knowledge of economic models to provide a foundation for understanding the issues that affect medical care and policy (Henderson, 2005).

3. It is important to strike a balance between incremental benefits and costs.

Decision making is seldom based on an all-or-nothing situation—it usually involves tradeoffs. For example, if we are to spend more on MRIs, then we need to spend a little less on mental health services. This chapter provides a gentle introduction to some of the basic economic concepts that underpin the more detailed and rigorous treatment of health economics in the remainder of the book.

beyond the point of equilibrium, the *MB* is not large enough to compensate the medical risk. The resources used to provide the excess care are better used elsewhere. Resources used in this wasteful fashion cannot be used in their next best alternatives, such as housing or transportation.

SUMMARY

Central tenets of economics can be summarized below:

1. Resources are relatively scarce related to wants. To strike a balance between scarce resources and unlimited

Key Words

- Market
- Equilibrium
- Scarcity
- Opportunity costs
- Marginal analysis
- Self-interest

- Supply and demand
- Competition
- Efficiency
- Market failure
- Marginal benefit
- Marginal cost

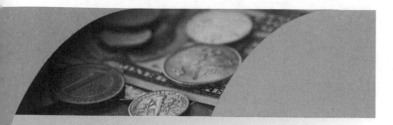

Questions

1. What is the appropriate role of economics in the study of the medical care sector? What are its strengths and what are the limitations?

2. Choices in medical care delivery can be made by the provider for the individual patient and by the policy maker who views the needs of an entire population of people. One way to choose among alternative treatments of care delivery models is through the determination of economic efficiency. Discuss the concept of efficiency.

REFERENCES

1. Fuchs, VR. (2005) Health care spending reexamined. *Annals of Internal Medicine,* 143:76–78.

2. Grossman, M. (1972) On the concept of health capital and the demand for health. *Journal of Political Economy,* 80(2):223–255.

3. Henderson, JW. (2005) *Health Economics and Policy,* 3d ed. Mason, Ohio: Thomson South-Western.

4. Reinhardt, UE, Hussey, PJ, and GF Anderson. (2002) Cross national comparisons of health care systems using OECD data 1999. *Health Affairs,* 21:169–181.

5. ——— (2004) U.S. health care spending in an international context. *Health Affairs,* 23:10–25.

6. Santerre, RE and SP Neun. (2004) *Health Economics: Theories, Insights and Industry Studies,* 3d ed. Mason, Ohio: Thomson South-Western.

BIO: JONATHAN FIELDING

Jonathan Fielding is a Professor of Health Services and Pediatrics and Co-Director of the UCLA Center for Healthier Children, Families and Communities at the University of California at Los Angeles. Dr. Fielding serves as Director of Public Health and Health Officer for Los Angeles County where he is responsible for the full range of public health activities for ten million county residents.

Dr. Fielding teaches Determinants of Health and participates as faculty lecturer in several of the Department courses. He received both his MD, MA (History of Science) and MPH from Harvard University, and his MBA from the Wharton School of Business Administration. His areas of expertise include the development of clinical preventive services guidelines, prevention economics and financing, and health promotion for children, adults, and families in community, clinical, and occupational settings. As the founding Co-Director of the Center for Health Enhancement, Education and Research at UCLA, he provided the first comprehensive university-based center to focus on clinical and worksite prevention opportunities. He formerly served as the Founding Board Member, Chairman of the Board, and member of the Executive Committee of The California Wellness Foundation, the largest U.S. foundation devoted to disease prevention and health promotion, and is among the 50 largest U.S. foundations. Further, he was a founding member of the U.S. Preventive Services Task Force and is Vice-Chair, Community Preventive Services Task Force. He is immediate past President of the American College of Preventive Medicine.

Dr. Fielding's awards include the Porter Prize, given for his national impact on improving the lives of Americans; and membership in the National Academy of Sciences Institute of Medicine. He is the author of over 150 original scientific articles and chapters, Editor of *Annual Review of Public Health,* and Associate Editor of the textbook, *Public Health and Preventive Medicine.*

Source: University of California Web site.

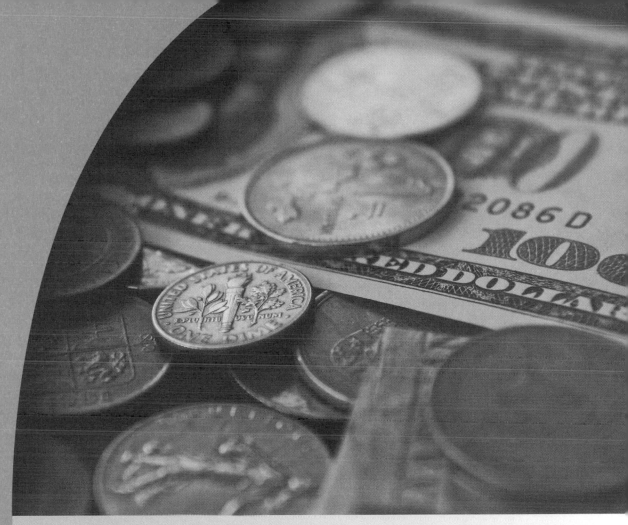

PART II

DEMAND

The Demand for Health

LEARNING OBJECTIVES:

In this chapter, you will learn about:

1. the determinants of individual and population health status.
2. the models for investment and consumption aspects of health.
3. the international comparisons of health among the United States and other developed countries.

GOOD HEALTH

Most of us probably find that it is obvious that everyone desires good health both for the sake of quality of life and because it contributes to our remaining productive and earning income. Yet a great deal of study has gone into determining what factors affect health and a formal model of investment in health is used by economists. We view health as a stock of capital that yields a stream of healthy days just as wealth is a stock of financial capital that yields a stream of income. In many cases, medical care is undertaken to gain more healthy days and it may therefore be interpreted as an investment in the stock of health. Anything that contributes to producing better health such as nutritious food, clean air, and exercise, can be considered health care (Johnson-Lans, 2006).

Improving health is not the only characteristic of health care that health economics takes into account. Many types of health care may impact on other aspects of a person's welfare— for example, providing reassurances or reducing anxiety about their state of health, whether or not their health has changed. Even when the main or sole purpose of health care is to improve health, the way in which it is provided may also be important—for example, the quality of meals that are provided during a stay in the hospital may be important to people even if that aspect has no impact on health. But for most types of health care, their most important and interesting characteristic is that they are intended to alter health, not that they are services provided by the healthcare industry (Morris et al., 2007).

This chapter presents a model of the demand for health with health care as an input for the production of health. It also takes into account that there may be negative consequences in the production of health. Formulating the basis for the demand for health provides the basis for the demand for health care—which is derived from the demand for health.

HEALTH AS A FORM OF HUMAN CAPITAL

The most important and powerful insight is that in addition to health care being an economic good, health itself can be thought of as a good, albeit one with special characteristics. It can be regarded as a fundamental commodity: one of the true

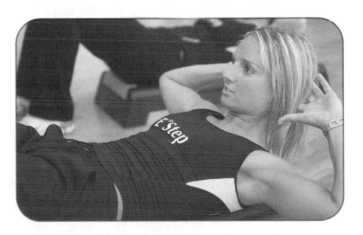

objects of people's wants and for which more tangible goods and services—such as health care—are simply a means to create it. This theory originates from the work of Becker (1965) and Grossman (1972), but it can be traced to 18th century economists such as Jeremy Bentham (1780), who wrote the "the relief of pain" as a "basic pleasure."

If it is accepted that health is a fundamental commodity, we can analyze the demand for improvements in health in very similar ways to the analysis of demand for other goods and services. A key difference is that because health is not tradable, it is not possible for it to be analyzed in the market framework (i.e., improvements in health cannot be purchased directly). Instead, we focus on the production of health as the key means in which people express their demand for it, which may involve the purchase of goods and services, thereby indirectly purchasing health improvements. Health care is therefore derived from the demand for health. Such analysis can be used for almost any goods or services, but it is of particular importance in health because the consumption of health care is usually not pleasurable, but is undertaken simply to improve health (Morris et al., 2007).

A model of the demand for health, developed in the 1970s by Michael Grossman, treats investment in health as a form of investment in **human capital** (Cuyler and Newhouse, 2000). The general model of human capital was originally developed by Gary Becker in his context of investment in education and it was logical to extend this to health (Becker, 1975).

Consider what is involved in the investment in any capital good. The analogy between health care and machine repair has often been made, so think about investing in a piece of machinery. A person might buy a machine in order to earn income as a consultant (e.g., if the machine is a computer). In this case the computer is a capital good. Or one might buy a computer to work and do pleasurable things, such as using the internet or playing games. In this case, the computer is also a capital good that provides a stream of services over time that has monetary value and value of utility or consumption aspects. The consumption aspects would be the joy of playing a favorite game on the weekend. If one only uses the computer for pleasure, it is still a capital good because it provides a stream of services over time (Johnson-Lans, 2006).

In order to improve the investment in a computer, some preventive maintenance is necessary, such as keyboard cleaning, virus protections, and so on. Sometimes, costly repairs are needed, such as a drive failure. In this case, the repair and maintenance of the computer is not unlike that of maintaining health. The amount of repairs needed by the computer depends on how it was treated. The routine maintenance and repairs on the computer are performed to offset depreciation.

This is part of the gross investment to the computer over the life of the machine. Gross investment includes the cost of purchasing the computer and its upkeep (Johnson-Lans, 2006).

Grossman's Investment Model of Health

The principle contribution of Grossman's model is the distinction between health as an output (i.e., a fundamental commodity), which is a source of utility to people, and medical care as an input to the production of health. In Grossman's model, health is both demanded and produced by individuals. Health is demanded because it affects the total time available for the production of income and wealth and because it is a source of utility itself. Ill health reduces both our happiness and our ability to earn.

Health is modeled as being produced by individuals, using a variety of means such as diet, lifestyle choices, and medical care. How efficient people are in the production of health depends on their knowledge and education. Medical care is but one input to the production of health. Each individual is modeled as starting life with a 'stock' of health, which has characteristics similar to capital: health depreciates through time with age, but can also be increased through investments in time, effort, knowledge, or by seeking health care.

Grossman's model captures two important insights. First, health care is but one input in generating improvements in health: it is now widely accepted that medical care is not the major determinant of health. Second, individuals do not demand health care for its own sake. The utility received from consuming health care is not generated from health care, but from the improvements in health that result. Therefore, the demand for health care is a derived demand.

The investment model of health views the demand for health as being conditional on both the cost of health capital and the rate of depreciation of the health stock. As in the investment in a computer, or in any capital good that eventually wears out, the difference between the gross (total) and net investment depends on the rate at which the capital good wears out or depreciates.

The **marginal efficiency of capital** (MEC) is a measure of how much extra output can be produced with an extra unit of input. Figure 3-1 depicts the schedule of the MEC of health capital. It shows how much extra expenditure is required to produce an additional unit of health stock. One measures the stock of health capital on the horizontal axis and the costs along the vertical axis. The MEC curve slopes downward because additional units of investment are assumed to yield smaller marginal improvements in the production of health. In other words, assume that the production of health is subject to **diminishing marginal returns**. H_i and H_{i+1} are two levels of

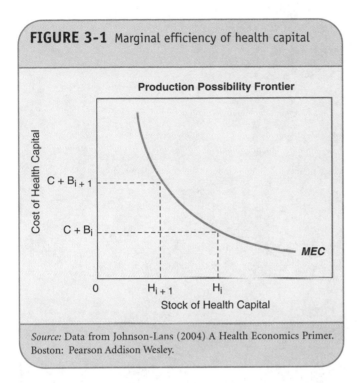

FIGURE 3-1 Marginal efficiency of health capital

Production Possibility Frontier

Source: Data from Johnson-Lans (2004) A Health Economics Primer. Boston: Pearson Addison Wesley.

health stock chosen by an individual at different levels of costs of health. The total cost of producing any health stock includes the cost of offsetting depreciation and the cost of incremental units of health stock, represented by C (Johnson-Lans, 2006).

One can think of the MEC schedule as the demand curve for health. It can also be seen as a production function for health because it relates inputs and the output of the stock of health. Once we know the MEC schedule, it is possible to know the level the individual will choose to produce. A rational person will invest additional resources in the production of health to the point where the value of additional degrees of healthiness is just equal to the marginal cost of producing it.

The MEC schedule is specific to an individual. The location of the MEC schedule depends on a person's initial stock of health at the beginning of the time period. An individual with a lower endowment of health will require more inputs to achieve the same health stock as an individual with a higher initial endowment. In that case, the MEC curve will be located to the left of the one that describes someone who begins life in a healthier state. The model does not assume that a given increase in inputs into the health production function will generate the same marginal improvement in different people (Johnson-Lans, 2006).

The Wage Effect

We treat the change in the wage rate as a shift in the MEC schedule because it changes the return from the stock of health.

It does so because the wage rate measures an individual's market efficiency (the rate in which healthy days are converted into monetary earnings), and also the opportunity cost of nonmarket time, as measured by the earnings foregone per hour or day. A stock of health is a better investment for high-wage earners because the individual's healthy working hours yield more income and the opportunity cost of his or her nonmarket time is also greater (Johnson-Lans, 2006).

The Consumption Model

For some purposes, it makes sense to shift to a model that focuses on the allocation of the budget (income) between investment in health and expenditure on consumer goods at any given time. In Figure 3-2, the straight line is the budget line. It shows the different combinations of health and consumption goods that one can purchase with a particular budget or income level. The quantity of goods that may be purchased from a budget depends on the prices of the goods. The slope of the budget line is determined by the relative prices of the goods, which are health and the consumer good.

U is an individual's **indifference curve**. Each indifference curve shows the various combinations of health and consumption goods that provide an individual with an equal amount of satisfaction or utility. A higher indifference curve represents a higher level of total utility. The standard assumption is that both the consumption good and health are subject to **diminishing marginal utility**: therefore, one can draw the indifference curves in the usual way, which is convex to the origin. Because one's productivity in the workplace is likely to be affected by one's health, investment in health could increase

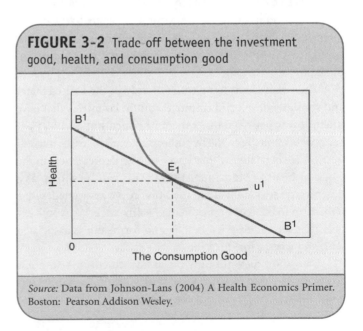

FIGURE 3-2 Trade-off between the investment good, health, and consumption good

Source: Data from Johnson-Lans (2004) A Health Economics Primer. Boston: Pearson Addison Wesley.

earnings to the extent that one might spend money on health care without reducing his consumption of other goods. Then there would be no tradeoff between the two. This diagram assumes that the effects of investment on health do not occur simultaneously. This diagram is meant to be a snapshot of a moment in time (Johnson-Lans, 2006).

ADDITIONAL FACTORS THAT AFFECT THE INVESTMENT IN HEALTH

Age

As one ages, it takes more resources to obtain or maintain a given stock of health. In contrast, older people are generally not charged higher prices for most consumer goods. In fact, some goods may be subject to senior citizen discounts, such as air travel, and some restaurant meals. Therefore, the relative pricing of producing health versus purchasing consumer goods tends to increase with age. The substitution effect (relative price effect) would encourage the substitution of other consumer goods for investment in health as one ages. In Figure 3-3, an increase in the relative price of health investment is shown by a decrease in the slope of the budget line from B_1B_1 to B_0B_1. This results in a new optimal combination of health and other goods as in E_1. A person with a very serious illness may decide it is not worth investing in the minimal health stock necessary to stay alive.

Education

We can use both the investment and consumption models to analyze the effects of education on the demand for health. Considerable evidence exists that more highly educated people are more efficient in the production of health. In the investment model, education shifts the MEC curve out to the right by raising the productivity of the inputs into the production of health.

The effect seems to be true not only in the United States and similarly developed countries, but in countries that have much lower per capita income and education and less advanced technologies. One hypothesis to explain this is that education is correlated with a lower rate of depreciation in the stock of health (Muurinen, 1982). This can be shown as a downward movement along the MEC curve associated with a reduction in the cost of producing health stock. We would expect that the increase in the demand for health is associated with an increase in education.

Education may not only make investment in health less costly, it may also be associated with different **time preferences**. Time preference is a term that refers to the extent to

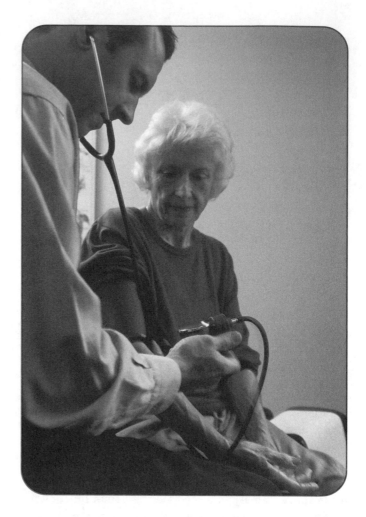

which people discount the future. The person who is preoccupied with the present ignores the future, that is, discounts it very heavily. Such a person is not likely to save or invest much in either education or health (Fuchs, 1982). Even if investment in education is correlated with investment in health, the effect of education on expenditure for health care is still an open question if greater efficiency in the production in health enables the use of fewer resources to attain any given level of health.

Lifestyle Effects of Wealth

The MEC curve may shift to the left as people become wealthier and consequently eating richer foods and lacking exercise. These are negative inputs into the production of health. Research has shown that there is a negative relationship between upturns in the economy and the level of healthiness in society (Grossman, 1972). In low-income countries, however, periods of prosperity would be expected to reduce malnutrition and lead to better health outcomes.

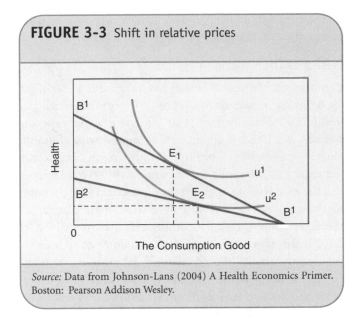

FIGURE 3-3 Shift in relative prices

Source: Data from Johnson-Lans (2004) A Health Economics Primer. Boston: Pearson Addison Wesley.

Chemical Dependency

In the case of addictive drugs, additional insight may be gained by utilizing both the investment and consumption models of health. Addiction might be viewed as shifting the marginal efficiency of health capital curve to the left, and it can also be viewed as causing a change in taste that would result in the substitution of the additive good for an expenditure on health. For example, one may reduce preventive care in order to afford more illegal drugs. A common view of drug addiction associates it with a very short time horizon in decision making, which is consistent with a diversion of resources away from investing in health to purchasing "utility-producing" addictive goods.

Following this reasoning, anything that increases the stock of health value will tend to reduce chemical dependency. In the case of addiction, better opportunities in the labor market which increase the value of healthy days, would tend to discourage chemical dependency (Johnson-Lans, 2006).

UNDERSTANDING THE INVESTMENT ASPECTS OF THE GROSSMAN MODEL

Grossman's theory is based on the idea of household and production. The true objectives are the fundamental commodities which are created within households by using time and market goods and services. The total time available can be used for either direct production of these commodities or for work to obtain income for market goods. For example, in creating the fundamental commodity related to eating, a household can have home-cooked, restaurant, take-out, or prepared meals. Each involves different combinations of the household's time and market goods. Analogously, health can be produced by diverse activities and goods such as exercise, diet, medical care, and lifestyle changes. The theory of health demand starts by assuming that for simplicity, people derive utility from two goods: health (H) and a composite of all other fundamental commodities (O), such that:

$$U = U(H,O)$$

Both H and O are sums over time, weighted by the person's time preference: different people have different preferences for when to obtain benefits, some being more impatient than others. H is therefore a weighted sum of the number of healthy days that the person enjoys over a lifetime. These healthy days derive from a person's stock of health (HS), thus greater health stock will lead to a greater number of healthy days. The health stock as a particular time (HS_t) is determined by the health stock in the previous period (HS_{t-1}) less any depreciation in health stock that has taken place over that period (d_t), plus any investment in health (I_t) that the person has undertaken, such that:

$$HS_t = HSt_{-1} - d_t + I_t$$

Health, in this way of thinking, is analogous to other types of capital, such as a machine. For example, one's health can depreciate over time due to excessive alcohol use or the effects of aging. But this can be offset by other investments that will improve health, such as lifestyle changes or medical care consumption. Both O and I are produced within the household, and we can define a production function for each of them. Production of O and I uses market goods, medical care (M) and all other market goods (X) respectively, and time spent on either in the production of health (T_H) or in the production of other goods (T_O). A third input to both is human capital, usually characterized as the level of education (E). The production functions are therefore:

$$I_t = I(M_t, T_H, E_t)$$
$$O_t = O(X_t, T_O, E_t)$$

It is assumed that a person will attempt to maximize their utility, but there are two constraints upon this—a time budget and an expenditure budget. The time budget (T) is fixed at 365.25 per year, where time is further constrained to time spent on working (T_W) and time spent being sick (T_S), such that:

$$T_t = T_{Ht} + T_{Ot} + T_{Wt} + T_{St}$$

The constraint on the expenditure budget is income, which depends on how much time is spent working and the wage rate (W). How much is spent depends on the costs of the market goods, M and X, and it is assumed that all income is spent, such that:

$$P_M \, xM + P_X \, xX = T_W \, xW$$

Both sides of the equation are in terms of present discounted values because they refer to a person's lifetime income and expenditures and are discounted at interest rate, r.

Maximization of the utility function, subjected to these constraints and taking into account the production function, leads to an equilibrium condition which can be interpreted as a person equalizing the marginal benefits of health capital and its marginal cost (Grossman, 1972).

EMPIRICAL EVIDENCE CONCERNING THE GROSSMAN MODEL

A large number of studies have been performed to determine the effects of age, schooling, and wealth on the demand for health (Muurinen, 1982). Researchers have constructed dynamic models to study how investing in health changes over the lifecycle and have introduced uncertainty into the investment model (Wagstaff, 1993). For example, if illness is defined as a state in which the stock of health falls beneath a critical level, the value of investing more in health stock is to reduce the likelihood of entering an illness state (Cropper, 1977). Therefore, health status results from a process in which the in-

dividual can only influence the probability of transitions from one health state to another (Zweifel and Breyer, 1997).

Critics of the Grossman Model

Critics of the Grossman model have argued that decisions about health care as part of a rational strategy for investing in health is belied by the facts. One argument is that expenditures on medical care are, in fact, correlated with ill health. Higher expenditures on health is simply a result of responses to negative shocks to the state of health. Others have posited that the great amount of uncertainty associated with the onset of illness makes it impossible to develop a rational plan for investing in health. Although it is undeniable that external shocks do alter the stock of health during the lifetime of an individual, dynamic models should be able to take this into account. Investment decisions are made in a world where there is uncertainty and lack of complete information (Johnson-Lans, 2006).

SUMMARY

Economists see the demand for health as an investment decision. Using this model, health care is not a consumer good, but an input into the production of the capital good—the stock of health. This chapter presented the widely-used model of the demand for health developed by Michael Grossman.

Key Words

- Human capital
- Marginal efficiency of capital
- Diminishing marginal returns
- Indifference curve
- Diminishing marginal utility
- Time preference

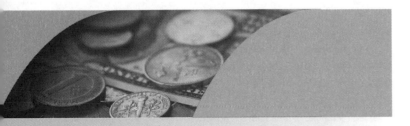

Questions

1. What factors make people more efficient in the production of stock of health?

2. Graphically show the change in demand for health when the wage rate increases.

3. What are the differences between the investment and consumption aspects of the investment in health?

4. How does aging affect the cost of acquiring health capital?

REFERENCES

1. Becker, GS. (1965) A theory of the allocation of time. *The Economic Journal*, 75:493–517.

2. ———— (1975) *Human Capital*. New York: National Bureau of Economic Research.

3. Bentham, J. An introduction to the principles of morals and legislation. In: Burns, JH and LHA Hart, eds. (1970), *The Collected Works of Jeremy Bentham*. London: Athlone Press.

4. Cropper, ML. (1977) Health, investment in health, and occupational choice. *Journal of Political Economy*. 85:275–294.

5. Cuyler, A and J Newhouse. (2000) *Handbook of Health Economics, Vol. 1*. Amsterdam: Elsevier.

6. Fuchs, V. Time preference and health: an exploratory study. In: Fuchs, V, ed. *Economics of Health*. Chicago: University of Chicago Press; 1982.

7. Grossman, M. (1972) On the concept of health capital and the demand for health. *Journal of Political Economy*, 80:223–255.

8. Johnson-Lans, S. (2006) *A Health Economics Primer*. Boston: Pearson Addison Wesley.

9. Morris, S, Devlin, N and D Parkin, (2007) *Economic Analysis in Health Care*. West Sussex, England: John Wiley & Sons, Ltd.

10. Muurinen, J. (1982) Demand for health: a generalized Grossman model. *Journal of Health Economics*, 1:5–28.

11. Wagstaff, A. (1993) The demand for health: an empirical reformation of the Grossman model. *Health Economics*, 2:189–198.

12. Zweifel, P and F Breyer. (1997) *Health Economics*. New York: Oxford University Press.

BIO: FRANK A. SLOAN

Frank A. Sloan earned his PhD at Harvard University and spent the first three years of his professional life as a research economist at RAND Corporation. While at RAND, he explored the implications and extensions of his dissertation on physicians' supply. He then went to the University of Florida and moved on to the Vanderbilt University in Tennessee, where he was the chair of the department and the Centennial Professor of Economics. Sloan then returned to his home state of North Carolina in his move to Duke University. Here, in addition to his appointment as the Alexander McMahon Professor of Health Policy and Management, he is also Professor of Economics and Senior Research Fellow at the Center for Demographic Studies.

Sloan has more than 200 publications in prestigious journals such as the *American Economic Review, Journal of Health Economics, Journal of the American Medical Association*, and the *New England Journal of Medicine*. He is also moving at a fast pace in publishing. He published 5 to 6 new articles per year and typically has about 10 to 15 papers under review at all times.

Sloan's early work focused on physicians and their work in the nation's hospitals. His article published in the *Journal of the American Medical Association* in 1983, "More Doctors: What will They Cost?", challenged the conventional wisdom that increasing physician supply would lower the cost of medical care. Even though economic theory suggested that increased supply for a given demand would lower costs, the physicians' market did not follow the same discipline as other markets.

In the mid 1980's, Sloan's research interests began to shift. With separate articles on medical malpractice and medical care for the elderly, both published in 1985, a gradual change in research emphasis began. Currently, his scholarship interests are in issues of tort liability and elder care.

Over the years, Sloan has been the principle investigator on more than 40 research grants, generating millions of dollars for his affiliated institutions. He is a member of the Institute of Medicine, of the National Academy of Science. Equally productive in the many roles he fills—teacher, writer, reviewer and consultant—his influence within health care circles knows no boundaries.

Source: Frank A. Sloan, curriculum vitae, Duke University Web site.
Health Economics and Policy, 2nd Edition. James W. Henderson. (Cincinnati, OH: South-western, 2002).

CHAPTER 4

The Demand for Health Care

LEARNING OBJECTIVES:

In this chapter, you will learn about:

1. the role of health care as an input to the production of health.
2. the responsiveness of demand for health care with respect to time, price, and income.
3. the relation of income and the demand for health care.

THE DEMAND FOR HEALTH CARE

Having established that we can construct a production function for health, we can consider the demand for health care, one of the inputs into the production function. Health care is different from the other inputs in the production of health in a number of ways. It has no utility apart from promoting health, unlike clothes, cars, and other consumption goods. Unlike other inputs, at least part of the demand for health care is unpredictable in that it is conditional on illness, and the level of expenditure on health care can be exorbitant when measured relative to household income and wealth. This chapter presents a model of the demand for health care, with health care as an input for the production of health (Johnson-Lans, 2006).

Anything that increases the demand for health should increase the demand for health care, other things being equal. For instance, higher wages, which make health days more valuable, should increase the demand for health and health care (Johnson-Lans, 2006). An exception would be when the time price of health care (e.g., the amount of time waiting for an appointment) is higher than the expected value of health care (Johnson-Lans, 2001).

The demand for health care also depends on the particular production function for health. Production functions are always constructed assuming a particular technology. Technological inputs in health care have increased the use of medical inputs in the production of health. They have also increased expectations about attainable health and therefore have increased the demand for health itself. This then increases the demand for health care.

The effect of education on the demand for health care is not as predictable. If education makes a person more efficient in producing health, an increased awareness of the value of good nutrition and prevention of disease will reduce the quantity of health care required to produce a given stock of health. Education can also increase the demand for health itself. The more educated will demand more health, but less health care, if the effect of education on the productivity of inputs into health outweighs the shift in the demand for health. Empirical research provides evidence of the ambiguity of education on the demand for health care (Wagstaff, 1986).

The effect of age on the demand for health care has been found to vary by type of health care required. For example, in an early study the demand for ambulatory care, such as seeing a physician during a given year, decreased significantly with age, but the demand for inpatient services and pharmaceuticals increased (Newhouse and Phelps, 1974). However, when the health status is included in the estimation including age on the demand for health care, age is no longer significant. It appears that the deterioration in health status that accompanies age, rather than age itself, increases the demand for health care (Zweifel, 1985).

The effect of insurance on the demand for health care is very important and will be addressed in more detail in future chapters. It primarily influences the price of health care, which is a movement along a given demand curve for health care.

In analyzing the demand for health care, it is important to take into account the concept of need when considering both the characteristics of health policy and an individual's consumption of health care. In most cases, need, rather than demand, dominates views about the aims of health services.

If you ask most people what determines their demand for health care, their answer will most likely be that they go to the doctor as needed. In contrast, the straightforward economics answer would be because they want to do so, which sounds peculiar because no one wants health care for its own sake (Evans, 1984). At face value, Grossman's theory (1972) provides a reconciliation of these two views because people want health improvements and demand care that will produce these improvements. However, need is more complicated than that. Need implies that there is an imperative to have health care because it will address health problems. People have limited knowledge about health problems and the care that will resolve them. In contrast, the usual assumption of economics is that in making demands, people are the best judges of their own wants (Johnson-Lans, 2006). Demand simply implies the willingness and ability to pay for health care.

Needs and demands can therefore be regarded as two very different ways of viewing matters, but considered together they give useful insights. Two extreme positions might arise. Sometimes there may be a demand with no need. People might be pessimistically mistaken about their health status or optimistically mistaken about the possibilities for improving it. In practice, the more important case is that there might be need where there is no demand, and if health services only responds to demand, then there is unmet need. Some of the unmet need will be due to deficiencies in information. Unmet needs may also be due to barriers to health care, such as supply factors (e.g., the availability of services to meet needs), and demand factors, such as prices and income levels which affect a person's ability to access services (Morris et al., 2007).

ASYMMETRY OF INFORMATION AND IMPERFECT AGENCY

A characteristic of the healthcare markets is uncertainty about diagnoses, available treatments, and effectiveness of those treatments (Arrow, 1963). Some of the uncertainty is irreducible, where neither the doctor nor the patient can know with certainty what the consequences of treatment will be (Pauly, 1978). This leads to the problem of unmet need. However, much of the uncertainty is one-sided: the consumer lacks the medical training and knowledge to make informed choices.

Information is itself an economic good. Obtaining information, for example, by engaging in consumer research to compare prices and qualities of alternative healthcare providers, or checking the relative costs and efficacies of alternative treatments, is worthwhile if the benefits exceed the costs. When the costs of obtaining information are too high, if information is highly specialized or difficult to obtain, or if the likely benefits are too low, consumers may choose to be rationally ignorant and to delegate decision making to the supplier of the services. Usually, the patient's contact with the doctor is when the doctor tells the patient what he or she should do (McGuire, 2001).

This relationship between doctor and patient is often presented as a principal-agent problem. The doctor is the agent acting on behalf of a principal, who is the patient, in making decisions about what health care to purchase. If doctors made these decisions in a manner fully consistent with patients' preferences, unaffected by the consequences for themselves, they would be acting as perfect agents—essentially making the healthcare decisions that the patients would do if they had access to the same information. Much of the economics literature has focused on the possibility that doctors either cannot or do not act as perfect agents. Specifically, the hypothesis of supplier-induced demand (SID) (Evans, 1984) purports that doctors engage in some persuasive activity to shift the patients' demand curve in or out depending on the physicians' self-interest (McGuire, 2001).

There is extensive theoretical and empirical literature on this subject. Early studies focused on testing the effects of increased availability of doctors on the utilization of health care. A problem with this literature is that many of the findings may be consistent with a noninducement model of how utilization is determined (Rice, 1998; Morris et al., 2007). In general, it

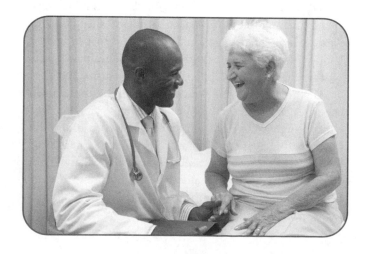

seems that there is no way in which observed movements in prices and quantities can prove inducement. Of course, this also means that there is no data to disprove it. However, some findings are clear: a comprehensive review of the literature demonstrates that physicians do respond to financial incentives and they do appear to influence demand and do so partly in response to self interest (McGuire, 2001). Even with this research, the definitive understanding of supplier-induced demand remains elusive. To confirm whether patients are being induced to demand more services than they really want, we would need to know how much they would have demanded if they were as well informed as the physician. No such study has been conducted (Rice, 1998; Mooney, 1994).

Estimates of the Price Elasticity of Demand for Health Care

We measure the responsiveness of consumers to changes in the price of a good or service by the **price elasticity of demand**. When measuring the degree of elasticity, a coefficient of -3 is a higher degree of elasticity than that of -0.1, because the coefficient of -3 represents a 300 percent decrease in quantity demanded for a 100 percent increase in price, where as a coefficient of -0.1 reflects only 10 percent decrease in quantity demanded associate with a 100 percent increase in price. The formula for elasticity of demand with respect to price is as follows:

$$\frac{\% \ change \ in \ the \ quantity \ of \ health \ care \ demanded}{\% \ change \ in \ price \ of \ health \ care}$$

In general, goods and services which are close substitutes have higher price elasticities, and complementary goods and services have lower price elasticities. The demand elasticity for a good that constitutes a higher proportion of income is also generally higher because the increase in the price of the good or service requires curtailing more consumption expenditures on other goods. An example of this is the price elasticity of demand for very high cost medical procedures. In these cases, the patient may forego the technology if there is no insurance cost share (Johnson-Lans, 2006).

The highest price elasticity estimates observed are for those demanding hospital outpatient services and for nursing home services (-1.00 and $-0.73 - -2.40$, respectively). Nursing home services have substitutes in home care and family care services and these costs represent a high proportion of the budget, which is another reason why elasticities are higher for these services (Zweifel and Breyer, 1997).

Researchers have also estimated price-elasticity on sensitivity to variations in prices among physicians and hospital services. Physician visits range from $-1.75 - -5.07$, and hospital services range from $-.02 - -1.12$ (Johnson-Lans, 2006). These are called from specific demand elasticity that the lower number of substitutes for hospitals make the elasticity for hospital services lower than that for physician services. However, once a physician is chosen, this also limits the number of hospitals that the patient can utilize as well due to the limits on admitting privileges of physicians.

Time Costs and Price Elasticities

The time cost is the value of time used in a given activity. Estimates of the price elasticity of demand for any good or service that requires time will tend to be biased if one does not take into account the time and money costs as well. The time cost of consuming a healthcare service would be the time involved in waiting for the appointment, as well as the travel time. The total cost of services that require time will be higher for patient with higher wage rates because they have a higher opportunity cost of time. Any factor that increases the value of time will increase the opportunity cost of time. For example, when insurance pays for a portion of the market price of health care, the time component of the cost becomes relatively large as a component of total cost. Insurance coverage has been shown to make time a more important consideration in the decision about how much medical care to seek and which providers to use (Acton, 1973). Studies have found that time costs are more important than money costs in the healthcare decisions (Coffey, 1983).

AGGREGATE DEMAND FOR HEALTH CARE

Using healthcare spending per person as a proxy measure for aggregate demand, researchers have found that most of the variation in healthcare demand among countries can be explained using just one variable: the country's income, generally measured as GDP per capita. It is clear that there is a positive relation between income and the demand for health care: the richer the country, the greater the demand for health care.

An influential paper on this issue by Newhouse (1977), using simple linear regression analysis in 13 countries, found that GDP per capita of a country explains 92 percent of the variance in the level of spending among the countries. These original findings and conclusions were the catalyst for vast literature reexamining the determinants of healthcare spending. More recently, contributions to the literature have focused on econometric issues arising from time series and panel data properties of the data sets used, testing for unit roots, and cointegration. The results have variously either been confirmed (Bloomqvist and Carter, 1997; Roberts, 1998) or contradicted (McCoskey and Selden, 1998). A review of the literature by

Gerdtham and Jonssen (2001) suggests that the most likely reason for the differences in results is differences in methods. They conclude that further research is required to provide a definitive answer.

HEALTH CARE: A NORMAL, SUPERIOR, OR INFERIOR GOOD?

A **normal good** is a good for which income elasticity is positive but less than one. This means that if income increases by a given percentage, the quantity of the good consumed increases, but at a lower percentage than associated with the income increase. If the percentage increase in the quantity consumed is greater than the associated percentage increase in income, the good is called a **superior good**. If the percentage increase in the quantity consumed is less than the associated percentage increase in income, the good is called an **inferior good**.

The answer to whether health care is a normal, superior, or inferior good, differs depending on whether we look at studies based on individual responses or those utilizing aggregate data. A number of studies in the 1960s through 1990s provides estimates of income elasticities for health care based on survey data derived from individual responses. A review of these studies shows consensus that most health care services have coefficients of income elasticity that are positive and in the r range of 0–1, and can be classified as normal goods. By contrast, studies using macroeconomic data do yield considerably higher income elasticity coefficients for health care. A wide range of studies have generally found health care to be a superior good. This is true for both industrialized and developing countries (Scheiber, 1990).

SUMMARY

The demand for health care depends on age, education, income, and health status. The demand for health care is generally sensitive to price and income, but price elasticities have values ranging between 0 to -1. Health care for which substitutes exist have higher elasticities than those with fewer substitutes, such as an acute care hospitalization. The association between income and the amount of health care utilized shows that health care can be a normal good when studies are based on individual responses. However, the macroeconomic data that compare country-wide aggregates in income and health-care spending show that health care is a superior good. This is true for industrialized nations and comparisons between those nations and developing countries.

Key Words

- Price elasticity of demand
- Normal good
- Superior good
- Inferior good

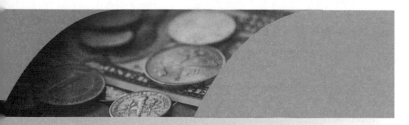

Questions

1. How would you expect the price elasticity of demand for health care to vary with health status?

2. Would the demand for health care increase or decrease with an improvement in educational attainment in the community? Explain.

3. Compare the time-price elasticity of demand if people reduce their physician visits by 20 percent when the travel time to get the nearest physician is from 15–45 minutes.

REFERENCES

1. Acton, JP. (1973) *Demand for Health When Time Prices Vary More than Money R-1189-OEO/NYC*. Santa Monica, CA: Rand Corporation.

2. Arrow, KJ. (1963) Uncertainty and the welfare economics of medical care. *The American Economic Review*, 53:941–973.

3. Bloomqvist, A and RAL Carter. (1997) Is health care really a luxury? *Journal of Health Economics*, 16:207–229.

4. Coffey, RM. (1983) The effect of time price on the demand for medical services. *The Journal of Human Resources*, XVIII:422.

5. Evans, R. (1984) *Strained Mercy: The Economics of Canadian Health Care*. Toronto: Butterworths.

6. Gerdtham, U and B Jonnsen. (2001) International comparisons of health care expenditures. In: Cuyler AJ and JP Newhouse, eds. *Handbook of Health Economics*, Vol. 1A. Amsterdam: North-Holland.

7. Grossman, M. (1972) On the correct concept of health capital and the demand for health. *Journal of Political Economy*, 80:223–255.

8. Johnson-Lans, S. (2001) Life style effects on the demand of college educated women for preventive care. Vassar College Working Paper Series.

9. Johnson-Lans, S. (2006) *A Health Economics Primer*. Boston: Pearson Addison Wesley.

10. McCoskey, S and TM Selden. (1998) Health care expenditure and GDP: panel data unit root test results. *Journal of Health Economics*, 17:369–376.

11. McGuire, T. Physician agency. In: Cuyler AJ and JP Newhouse, eds. *Handbook of Health Economics*, Vol 1A. Amsterdam: North Holland; 2001.

12. Mooney, G. (1994) *Key Issues in Health Economics*. New York: Harvester Wheatsheaf.

13. Morris, S, Devlin, N and D Parkin. (2007) *Economic Analysis in Health Care*. West Sussex, England: John Wiley & Sons, Ltd.

14. Newhouse, JP. (1977) Medical care expenditures: a cross-national survey. *Journal of Human Resources*, 12:115–124.

15. ———— and CE Phelps. New estimates of price and income elasticities of medical care services. In: *The Role of Health Insurance in the Health Services Sector*. New York: National Bureau of Economic Research; 1974.

16. Pauly, MV. Is medical care different? In: Greenburg A, ed. *Competition in the Health Care Sector: Past, Present and Future*. Colorado: Aspen Systems; 1978.

17. Rice, T. (1998) *The Economics of Health Reconsidered*. Chicago: Health Administration Press.

18. Roberts, J. (1998) Spurious regression problems in the determination of health care expenditure: a comment on Hitiris. *Applied Economics Letters*, 7:279–283.

19. Scheiber, GJ. (1990) Health care expenditures in major industrialized countries, 1960–1987. *Health Care Financing Review*, 11:159–167.

20. Wagstaff, A. (1986) The demand for health: some new empirical evidence. *Journal of Health Economics*, 5:195–237.

21. Zweifel, P. The effect of aging on the demand and utilization of medical care. In: C. Tilquin, ed. *Systems Science in Health and Social Services for the Elderly and Disabled*. Toronto: Pergamon Press; 1985.

22. ———— and F Breyer. (1997) *Health Economics*. New York: Oxford University Press.

BIO: MARK V. PAULY

Mark V. Pauly's career was launched by his 1968 article in the *American Economic Review*, "The Economics of Moral Hazard." After receiving his PhD in 1967, this paper catapulted him into the epicenter of health economics. This work has become essential reading on the effect of health insurance on healthcare utilization and costs.

After brief academic appointments at Northwestern University and his alma mater, the University of Virginia, Pauly moved to the University of Pennsylvania's Wharton School where he became the executive director of the Leonard Davis Institute (LDI) of Health Economics. Founded in 1967, the LDI has maintained a commitment to health services research and education in an interdisciplinary setting. Pauly is the LDI Senior Fellow and Professor of Health Care Systems, Public Policy and Management, Insurance and Risk Management, and Economics. He is also the Bendheim Professor and vice dean and director of doctoral programs.

Pauly has made an unbelievable contribution to health economics literature. With more than 100 books, articles, and monographs in print, he research interests encompass medical economics and the role of markets in health care, national healthcare policy, and health insurance. In addition, he is a member of the editorial boards of the *Journal of Health Economics* and the *Journal of Risk and Uncertainty*, and an elected member of the Institutes of Medicine of the National Academy of Science.

Pauly's belief that the incentive structure can shape both the behavior of patients and providers has resulted in his teaming with John C. Goodman, Director of the National Center for Policy Analysis in publishing the article, "Tax Credits for Insurance and Medical Savings Accounts" in Spring 1995 issue of *Health Affairs*. This innovative approach to healthcare reform recommends the use of tax credits, medical savings accounts, and high-deductible insurance to improve efficiency and equity in the healthcare sector.

If the essential ingredients for making good choices are knowledge and inquiry, Pauly has advanced our ability to make enlightened choices through his outstanding contribution to health economics and the economics of insurance.

Source: Mark V. Pauly, curriculum vitae.
Health Economics and Policy, 2nd Edition. James W. Henderson. (Cincinnati, OH: South-western, 2002).

The Market for Health Insurance

THE INSURANCE MARKET

People buy insurance because they are risk-averse. Buying insurance allows a person to pay a certain known amount in order to transfer the risk of a much larger expenditure (in the case of an adverse event) to an insurer, known as a third party payer. Firms sell insurance because they are paid to assume a risk that can be managed by spreading it over a large pool of the insured. Insurance markets exist where consumers are willing to pay enough to transfer risk to induce insurance companies to assume the risk. This chapter examines the characteristics of insurance markets and, together with Chapter 5, considers the unique aspects of the insurance market (Johnson-Lans, 2006).

There are a number of types of risk associated with health. There is the risk to one's health and life associated with illness or disease. There is the additional risk that if one undertakes treatment, it may or may not cure or alleviate symptoms of disease. There are also the costs associated with the treatments of illness and disease. A person can take action to reduce the risk of illness such has getting vaccines, avoiding unhealthy environments, and leading a healthy lifestyle. One cannot insure against bad health outcomes, though. However, people can insure themselves against some or all of the financial loss associated with the treatment of illness by buying health insurance policies (Johnson-Lans, 2006).

People don't generally self-insure by saving money when well to use in times of illness. Much of this is due to the fact that people cannot save enough for catastrophic illnesses. Even people with extensive wealth buy insurance due to the fact that most people are "risk-averse."

Economists define risk aversion as a characteristic of people's utility functions. Consumers' attitudes toward risk depends on the marginal utility of an extra dollar that may be different in different ranges of wealth. If the marginal utility of wealth decreases as wealth increases, there is a small probability of a smaller amount of wealth when the probability weighted or expected value of the alternatives is equal. That is a situation of risk aversion. Risk-loving people gamble when gambling involves an unfair bet. Betting on lotteries would be rational behavior in a range of wealth when the marginal utility of an extra dollar is increasing. In general, it is assumed that people are more likely to buy insurance to cover low-probability events involving large losses than high-probability events that are associated with small losses, and they are more likely to buy lottery tickets when there is a low probability of winning a large amount (Johnson-Lans, 2006).

Setting Insurance Premiums

Insurance is a mechanism for assigning risk to a third party. It is also a mechanism for pooling risk over a large group of insured persons. The price that an insurance company charges for an insurance policy, or premium, is based on the expected payout (amount paid out on average for a large group of insured persons), plus administrative costs, reserve funds, and profits or surpluses of the insured company. As a result, premiums charged generally exceed the fair value of the risk that the insurance company has assumed, where the fair value is the expected payout.

The part of the insurance premium that exceeds the fair value of the insurance is called the loading fee. It is theoretically correct to think of the load, not the premium, as the price of insurance. The price of insurance is the cost of transferring risk. Particularly when comparing different insurance policies, it is convenient to express the loading fee as a percentage based on the ratio of premium to expected payout:

$$L = 100 \times ((premium/E) - 1),$$
$$where\ E = probability\ of\ illness \times treatment\ costs.$$

Suppliers of insurance will be more willing to enter market situations where they can make a reasonable estimate of what their payouts will be, or where they can assess the degree of risk they are assuming. They will also be more willing to insure risky events about which the probability of occurrence is better known (Johnson-Lans, 2006).

Experience versus Community Rating

One common method of pricing insurance is **experience rating**. This occurs when insurance companies base premiums on past levels of payouts, which is often done in the case of car or homeowners' insurance. Drivers who have been in an auto accident will find their rates increased. In the case of health insurance, age and preexisting conditions may be good predictors of future utilization of healthcare services and may be used to determine premiums (Johnson-Lans, 2006).

Community rating applies when each member of an insurance pool pays the same premium per person or per family for the same coverage. Community rating is inefficient in the sense that the price of insurance to an individual subscriber does not reflect the marginal costs of that individual to the insurer. However, the tradeoff between equity and efficiency is usually also considered. Not only more societies support some intertemporal risk sharing, but also some societies favor sharing of risk between health (or low-risk) and ill (high-risk) individuals (Johnson-Lans, 2006).

Moral Hazard

Moral hazard refers to the phenomenon of a person's behavior being affected by his or her insurance coverage. Moral hazard is known to exist is in all types of insurance markets. For example, people may be more careless with property that is insured. The main way that moral hazard comes into play in the health insurance market is through an increase in demand for healthcare services utilized.

Moral Hazard and the Structure of Health Insurance Contracts

The reason that moral hazard operates differently in the health insurance market than in other insurance markets is that health insurance contracts differ from most other forms of insurance. Instead of paying a sum of money to the insured in the case of an adverse event, they reduce the price of the health care associated with the adverse event or illness.

Moral hazard, in the context of the health insurance market is illustrated in Figures 5-1a and b. An individual's demand for health care when he or she has no insurance is denoted by D_0D. If insurance pays 100 percent of the healthcare bill, the demand curve will shift to D_2D, because the individual treats the service as free. D_1D depicts a situation where insurance covers only part of the charges for the service. The price on the axis is the full market price of care, as shared by the insurer and the insured. Therefore, the insured has not had a shift in demand for healthcare services per se, but is responding to the de facto decline in price that results from the insurance company paying all or part of the medical bill (Johnson-Lans, 2006).

Some degree of moral hazard exists when the price elasticity of demand for covered healthcare services is greater than zero. In theory, the problem of moral hazard should be greater in the case of policies covering a broader range of services, including more discretionary or elective ones, because the price elasticity of demand for these services is believed to be higher. The degree of moral hazard accounts for the patient's insurance status in making decisions about how much treatment to prescribe.

Major healthcare services contracts also differ from most types of insurance in that they generally cover more than just unlikely catastrophic events, also fulfilling a function analogous to that of a service contract on an automobile. For example, they also include reimbursement for annual physical exams, vaccinations, treatment for chronic conditions, and various types of routine tests. The demand for these services is neither unpredictable nor does it usually entail catastrophic levels of expenditures (Johnson-Lans, 2006).

Cost Sharing to Offset Effects of Moral Hazard

Deductibles. A deductible is a level expenditure that must be incurred before any benefits are paid out. Homeowners' insurance policies generally have a deductible per event. The difficulty in deciding what is a separate event in the case of health problems makes this kind of deductible impractical in health

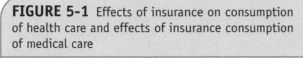

FIGURE 5-1 Effects of insurance on consumption of health care and effects of insurance consumption of medical care

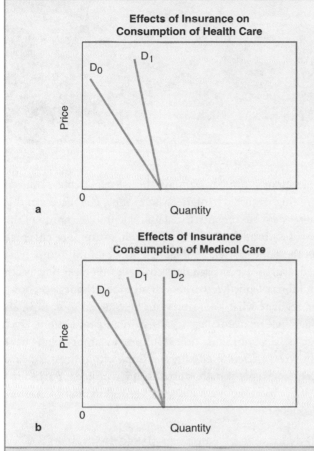

Effects of Insurance on Consumption of Health Care

Source: Data from Johnson-Lans (2004) A Health Economics Primer. Boston: Pearson Addison Wesley.

care. Health insurance policies generally have yearly deductibles, which is less effective in removing moral hazard. As is typical of all kinds of insurance, the load factor tends to be higher on health insurance policies with low deductibles because administrative costs constitute a higher proportion of the total cost of the policy to the insurer.

Coinsurance. Coinsurance is the proportion of the total expenditure that is paid by the insured. Coinsurance helps to reduce the moral hazard factor for the insured that have spent more than their deductible because health care is not free to them.

Use of Usual, Customary Fees to Limit Payments. It has become common practice for insurance policies that reimburse on the basis of fee-for-service to limit payment for covered services to customary or usual fee within given geographic markets. If a provider charges higher-than-customary fees, the insured is responsible for the balance of the fee, as well as the copayment on the covered portion. It discourages the consumer insensitivity to price. This may be another manifestation of moral hazard.

Managed Care. Managed care is a catch-all phrase that describes a variety of different kinds of insurance instruments. Care is actually managed or rationed using such mechanisms as "gatekeepers," who are primary care physicians that make all referrals to specialists, limit coverage to service providers with whom the insurance company has a contractual agreement, and require precertification or approval from the insurance company before services are rendered. Controls are on the supply side as well as the use of risk-sharing arrangements with providers of health care.

Stop-Loss Provisions. Many policies also have annual limits on out-of-pocket expenditures (per person or per family) that must be borne by the insured. This is called a stop-loss provision. After the insured has paid out an amount equal to the stop-loss threshold, the insurance company pays 100 percent of additional coverage to healthcare expenses during the year. This increases moral hazard for those with annual level of expenditures that exceed the stop-loss limit.

Adverse Selection

Adverse selection exists when people with different health-related characteristics than the average person increase the amount of health insurance purchased. People know more about their own health status than insurers, and this inequality of information is the basis for risk to insurers due to adverse selection.

In the health insurance market, high risk people are those with more severe health problems than the average person. These people would be overrepresented in the insurance markets, particularly those markets with more inclusive policies. This would drive up the premium because the high risk persons would use more health care and drive off those with better health from buying the insurance policies. The existence of adverse selection is an argument for a single payer plan because those with higher risk would not be able to pick their insurance plan and everyone would be in the same insurance pool (Johnson-Lans, 2006).

Insurers' Responses to Selection Problems

Insurers engage in positive selection, where the companies structure coverage to both avoid adverse selection and also to attract lower-than-average risk subscribers. Marketing efforts may be concentrated in communities known to have younger and healthier subscribers. In some cases, insurance companies do not enter or limit participation in markets with large amounts of adverse selection. Because insuring groups of people has the effect of offsetting adverse selection, insurers often avoid the individual or direct pay insurance market.

The disappearance of insurance options due to the spiraling costs associated with adverse selection has been a serious problem in the market for individual direct pay policies in regions that require community rating. However, New York State's move in 1993 to require community rating for all insurance companies selling policies to individuals or small groups does not appear to have had much effect. A study found no difference in the percentage change in individuals or small groups covered by health insurance in New York before and after this reform when compared to Connecticut and Pennsylvania, which did not impose community rating in the small group and individual markets (Buchmueller and DiNardo, 1999).

Offsetting Adverse Selection

Some economists have questioned whether health insurance markets can reach equilibrium, given the role of adverse selection (Rothschild and Stiglitz, 1976). This is because consumers no longer have much of the information advantage in choosing the best package of insurance to cover their future expenditures.

The condition necessary for insurance markets to function, even with the problems of adverse selection, was summarized 25 years ago. It is still relevant today: neither insurance firms nor their customers have to be perfectly informed about the differences in risk properties that exist among individuals. What is required is that individuals with different risk properties differ on some characteristic that can be linked to the purchase of insurance and that there is some way that an insurance company can discover the link (Rothschild and Stiglitz, 1976).

EMPLOYER-BASED INSURANCE

Advantages of Employer-Based Insurance

The majority of nonretired Americans who have private health insurance are covered by group policies that are part of employer contracts. Employer-based insurance has dominated the markets since the 1950s, when price controls on wages made fringe benefits an important part of increasing worker compensation. Group insurance is important for offsetting adverse selection. This is one of the reasons for its success. Community rating applies within the employment group, which results in some degree of risk sharing. Economies of scale in administrative rates are lower than those for individual or direct pay policies (Johnson-Lans, 2006).

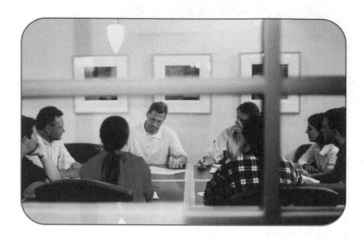

Insurance companies may still use experience rating to charge higher prices to higher-risk groups. The success of this strategy depends on both the stability within the group of the insured and the duration of the group's insurance coverage with the same carrier. Federal law now prohibits employer-based insurance from excluding coverage for preexisting health conditions even when workers change jobs. It does not, however, regulate what premiums can be charged to groups, although state regulatory agencies may impose restrictions. Over time, as selections and choices among insurance plans have come to be offered to employee groups within firms, adverse selection has emerged, thus proving it is a problem not limited solely to the individual and small group market (Johnson-Lans, 2006).

Disadvantages of Employer-Based Insurance

When health insurance is tied to employment, job loss involves the risk of losing access to affordable health insurance. The consolidated Omnibus Budget Reconciliation Act of 1985 (COBRA) requires employers to offer former employees an option of purchasing their former group health insurance coverage for up to 18 months after termination of employment. This provides only a temporary solution and may be unaffordable because the employee must pay the entire premium plus a two percent fee (Johnson-Lans, 2006).

The tying of health insurance to employment reduces labor mobility and results in what is considered to be job lock. Research concludes that employer-provided insurance has reduced labor mobility by about 25 to 30 percent (Gruber, 2000). The **Health Insurance Portability and Accountability Act (HIPAA) of 1996** addresses part of the problem by making it illegal for insurers to exclude any employee from a group plan on the basis of health-related factors or past claims history. However, it may not be possible to find a new job with health benefits and for an individual who has left employment due to ill health, it may not be possible to secure employment at all. In addition, employers may be unwilling to hire a worker whose preexisting conditions may drive up the group health insurance premiums (Johnson-Lans, 2006).

Tax Treatment of Employer-Based Health Insurance

Under federal and state income tax law, health insurance premiums paid by employers as part of the workers' compensation package have been tax-free income to employees and tax-deductible labor costs for firms since 1954. This has led to worker preferences for higher proportions of their compensation packages in the form of health insurance, because firms can offer workers' compensation that represents more after-tax benefits than a cash wage package costing the firm an equal amount. There is further saving to firms and workers in the form of payroll tax (FICA) exclusions on the portion of compensation paid in health insurance premiums rather than wages (Johnson-Lans, 2006).

The income-tax free status of employer-based insurance has income distribution effects. Because the federal income tax is progressive, workers with higher wages and salaries who pay higher marginal tax rate receive a larger subsidy.

OPTIMAL INSURANCE CONTRACTS

Constructing an optimal insurance policy is challenging when considering the issue of adverse selection. Where there is a menu of health insurance plans available, the less healthy people will be attracted to the more generous plans. A common form of partial risk sharing requires the more generous plans to charge only for the extra cost associated with the extra benefits. In this strategy, it is assumed that the health-related characteristics of members of different plans are the same on average. This method is often used for pricing employer-based insurance. Optimal insurance also needs to consider the degree of risk sharing between healthcare providers and insurers. Optimality requires a balance such that the providers neither provide more than medically appropriate nor withhold care. One problem in modeling the optimal insurance contract is that the degree of moral hazard may vary by type of illness or type of healthcare service. This may lead to very complicated insurance contracts with different degrees of copayments for different services (Johnson-Lans, 2006).

There are a wide variety of results associated with empirical research involving optimal insurance contracts. Estimates of optimal coinsurance rates vary from 25 to 58 percent. Estimates of the optimal stop-loss limits vary from $1000 to greater than $25,000. Using the RAND Health Insurance Experiment Data, Bloomqvist constructed an optimal policy that features coinsurance rates that vary by level of spending.

In this plan, up to an expenditure of $1000 out-of-pocket, one would pay a 27 percent coinsurance rate. Beyond that level, coinsurance rates would be reduced. When the out-of-pocket expenses rise above $30,000, the coinsurance rate is reduced to 5 percent (Cutler and Zeckhauser, 2000).

REIMBURSEMENT

The method of reimbursement relates to the way in which healthcare providers are paid for the services they provide. It is useful to distinguish between reimbursement methods because they can affect the quantity and quality of health care. We focus on methods for reimbursing hospitals.

Retrospective Reimbursement

Retrospective reimbursement at full cost means that hospitals receive payment in full for all healthcare expenditures incurred in some prespecified period of time. Reimbursement is retrospective in the sense that not only are hospitals paid after they have provided treatment, but also in that the size of the payment is determined after treatment is provided. Total reimbursement, p, is given either by:

$$P = WxAC$$

Or by:

$$P = Wx(SxI)$$

Where W = workload (e.g., number of cases treated), AC = average cost of service provided per case, s = number of services provided per case, and I = fee per item of service. Which model is used depends on whether the hospital is reimbursed for actual costs incurred or on a fee-for-service basis (Johnson-Lans, 2006).

In the actual costs model, hospital income depends on workload and actual costs incurred. In the fee-for-service model, reimbursement depends on workload and the services provided. It may be set by competition or by the third party payer. Because hospital income depends on the actual costs incurred or on the volume of services provided, there are few incentives to minimize costs. For example, hospitals might encourage excessively long lengths of stay or may over-order diagnostic tests (Johnson-Lans, 2006).

Prospective Payment

Prospective payment implies that payments are agreed upon in advance and are not directly related to the actual costs incurred. This does not mean that the hospital received the payment in advance, only that the size of the payment is determined in advance. Because payment is not directly related to the actual costs incurred, incentives to reduce costs are greater, but payers may need to monitor the quality of care provided and access to services. If the hospital receives the same income regardless of quality, there is a financial incentive to provide low-quality care for minimum effort and minimum cost.

Prospective reimbursement can take two forms. With global budgeting, the size of the budget paid to the hospital is set prospectively across the whole range of treatments provided. It is unrelated to the actual costs incurred and to workload. This provides a financial incentive to constrain total expenditure ($= WxAC$).

Global budgeting gives overall expenditure control to the third party payer, but because the way in which the global budget is distributed throughout the hospital is not specified, the allocation of the global budget within the hospital may not be efficient. The size of the global budget might be set historically with an additional adjustment made each year to account for inflation and changes in case mix, or it might be set according to a resource allocation formula based on the size of the need-weighted population served by the provider. In the latter case, the incentives of the global budget will depend on the precise components of the formula (Johnson-Lans, 2006).

With prospectively set costs per case, the amount paid per case (SxI) is determined before treatment is provided. By setting the costs per case prospectively, reimbursement is divorced from the costs incurred (AC) or the services provided per case (S), which generates incentives for the cost containment. Total reimbursement can still be increased by increasing workload. So, unlike global budgeting, this method does not provide overall expenditure control to the third party payer (Johnson-Lans, 2006).

An example of prospectively set costs per case is the diagnosis-related groups (DRGs) pricing scheme introduced by Medicare in 1984 and later used in other countries. Under this methodology, DRG payments are based on average costs per case in each diagnostic group derived from a sample of hospitals. Total reimbursement achieved by a hospital is given by:

$$P = Wx(DRG)$$

Where DRG is the DRG-based prospective payment.

The precise effect of this type of reimbursement will depend on the actual costs incurred by the hospital. If $DRG < AC$, hospitals will reduce AC until $DRG = AC$; hospitals have an incentive to minimize costs. If $DRG > AC$, hospitals will increase costs until $DRG = AC$. They will spend more on amenities in order to improve their competitive position in the healthcare market, which will cause AC to rise (Johnson-Lans, 2006).

Predicted effects of the DRG pricing method are cost shifting, patient shifting, and DRG creep. Cost shifting and patient shifting are ways of circumventing the cost-minimizing effects of DRG pricing. This is accomplished by shifting patients or some of the services provided to patients out of the DRG pricing method and into other parts of the system not covered by DRG pricing (e.g., shifting inpatient care to outpatient care, which is reimbursed retrospectively). DRG creep arises when hospitals deliberately or inadvertently classify cases into DRGs that carry a higher payment, indicating that they are more complicated than they really are. This might arise, for instance, when cases have multiple diagnoses (Johnson-Lans, 2006).

INTEGRATION BETWEEN THIRD PARTY PAYERS AND HEALTHCARE PROVIDERS

There are three different kinds of integration between third party payers and healthcare providers. First, the third party payer and provider are separate entities with separate aims and objectives. Second, there is selective contracting, with the third-party payer agreeing to steer individuals insured on their plans to selected providers, and, in turn, the selected providers charge lower prices to the insurers. Third, there is vertical integration in which the insurance provider and healthcare provider merge to become different parts of the same organization. Vertical integration means that a single organization provides health care in return for payment of an insurance premium. Because the two entities are parts of the same organization, they have common goals with respect to cost and quality of care. This is a key feature of managed care (Johnson-Lans, 2006).

Managed Care Organizations

Managed care organizations (MCOs) have arisen predominantly in the private health insurance sector in the United States as a means to control spiraling healthcare costs arising from the traditional private health insurance model (sometimes called the indemnity plan). Typically, health care is provided by an MCO to a defined population at a fixed rate per month. The payments made by individuals are lower than the direct out-of-pocket payment or indemnity plans. In return for lower premiums, enrollees are required to receive health care from a limited number of providers with whom the MCO has negotiated lower reimbursement rates. There are three broad types of MCOs, reflecting the extent of integration between third party payers and healthcare providers.

Preferred Provider Organizations

In return for payment of the insurance premium, preferred provider organizations (PPOs) provide insured individuals with two options when they require treatment. First, they can use the PPO's providers—those with which it contracts selectively in return for lower reimbursement rates. By using a preferred provider, individuals face lower user charges, and so the reduced costs of care with the preferred provider are passed on to the consumer. Alternatively, individuals may choose to use a different provider outside of the network of preferred providers, but will incur higher user charges. Patients can choose freely because there are no gatekeepers restricting the choices, however there is a clear financial incentive to stay within the network of preferred providers.

Health Maintenance Organizations

In its simplest form the main feature of a health maintenance organization (HMO) is that the insurance company and the healthcare provider vertically integrate to become different parts of the same organization. The HMO provides health care to the individual in return for a fixed fee, therefore combining the role of the third party payer and the healthcare provider. Health maintenance organization members are assigned a primary care provider who serves as a gatekeeper responsible for authorizing any health care provided. The individual must pay the additional charge for any treatment not authorized.

There are four broad types of HMOs, reflecting different relationships between the third party payer and the healthcare provider. In the staff model, the HMO employs physicians directly. In the group model, the HMO contracts with a group practice of physicians for the provision of care. In the network model, the HMO contracts with a network of group practices. In the case of independent practice associations, physicians in small independent practices contract to service HMO members.

Point-of-Service Plans

Point-of-Service (POS) plans are a mixture of PPOs and HMOs. As with the PPOs, in return for payment of an insurance premium, patients have two options when they require treatment: use the preferred provider network and pay lower charges; or use the non-networked providers on less favorable financial terms. Unlike PPOs, however, POS plans employ primary care physician gatekeepers who authorize any health care provided by the preferred provider network. In this way, POS plans are like HMOs (Morris et al, 2007).

OPTIONS FOR HEALTHCARE FINANCING

The exposition in this section draws heavily from Mossialos et al. (2002).

Private Health Insurance

This type of insurance has all the main features of the basic health insurance model developed in the first part of the chapter. Individuals enter into contracts with insurance providers voluntarily and pay premiums out-of-pocket or are paid by their employers as part of their salary package or both. **Private health insurance** is usually supplied by providers for profit, though it can also be offered by public bodies or by nonprofit organizations. The size of the insurance premium is usually based on the risk status of the insured individual. Patients may be required to pay user charges, in the form of copayments or deductibles to cover all or part of the costs of their health care.

Private insurance can be substitutive, when it provides the only form of insurance cover for the individual; complementary, when it provides coverage for health care that is excluded or not fully covered by compulsory insurance systems; or supplementary, when its role is to increase subscriber choice of provider and improve access. Private health insurance can be provided via indemnity plans or MCOs.

Social Insurance

Here, workers, employers, and government all contribute to the financing of health care by paying into a **social insurance** fund. Payments by employees can be fixed, or related to the size of their income, but not to their individual risk. Many countries finance their social insurance funds by means of a payroll tax, each firm paying an amount depending on the number of people they employ. The social insurance funds are usually independent of direct government control.

Membership in social insurance funds may be assigned according to occupation or region of residence, or individuals may be free to choose a fund. Children are covered through their parents' funds, and husbands and wives who do not work are covered by their spouses' funds. Contributions can be made into social insurance funds for retired and unemployed individuals either by the state, or via pension funds and unemployment funds.

HEALTH INSURANCE AND THE CONSUMPTION OF HEALTH CARE

It was demonstrated that health insurance operates to increase the quantity of health care demanded by lowering the effective price to consumers. The magnitude of the effect will depend on how much the policy reduces the out-of-pocket payment below the market price and the price elasticity of demand for health care. There is a potential problem in that the amount of insurance coverage people choose may not be independent of their demand for health care. The RAND Health Insurance Experiment provided estimates that are free from this bias; and the study design allows estimation of the effects of marginal rates of insurance coverage on the quantity of health care consumed. The RAND study found a range of coinsurance elasticity estimates for health care centering on −0.2 (Newhouse, 1988). This means that when coinsurance rates change by 10 percent, the quantity of health care utilized changes by 2 percent. This estimate is widely used in economic studies (Zweifel and Manning, 2000).

Insurance Coverage and Time Costs

When insurance coverage lowers the monetary costs of healthcare services to people, the time cost becomes a more important component of total cost. This will tend to increase the time-price elasticity of demand for health care, with the result being that consumers may shift to using healthcare services that have higher monetary costs, but less time costs (e.g., waiting time or travel time). Increases in wages or salaries increase the opportunity cost of time, which will lead to a tendency to substitute away from time-intensive health care. To the extent that insurance coverage is positively correlated with earnings, the substitution from time-intensive healthcare services to more expensive services will be enhanced (Johnson-Lans, 2006).

Insurance Coverage and the Market Price of Health Care

More extensive insurance coverage on the part of a community will tend to increase the quantity of health care that will be consumed at a given market price. This implies that there will be a shift in demand. Figures 5-2a and b show that a hypothetical increase in a community's demand for health care will depend on the change in its market price, as well as the change in insurance coverage. This also depends on the nature of the supply of services in the market. The supply curve is upward sloping as the change in the price of health care causes a rise in the quantity of health care supplied. Over time, the out-of-pocket prices of health care for the community will rise as the market price of health care rises. Insurance companies will also experience higher payouts, and they will respond by raising premiums charged for the same coverage or by holding premiums constant and reducing coverage (Johnson-Lans, 2006).

Health policy analysts are interested in what happens to the community's total expenditures on health care as insurance coverage increases. In Figures 5-2a and b, the community's expenditure on health care, not including insurance costs, is represented by $P_1 x Q_1$—before expansion of insurance coverage, and $P_2 x Q_2$ after demand shifts outward. Total expenditures on health care rises with an increase in insurance coverage even though there may be little change in total out-of-pocket expenditures. A full consideration of healthcare expenditures should also include an analysis of the expenditure on insurance. For instance, research based on the RAND Health Insurance Experiment data estimates that only ten per-

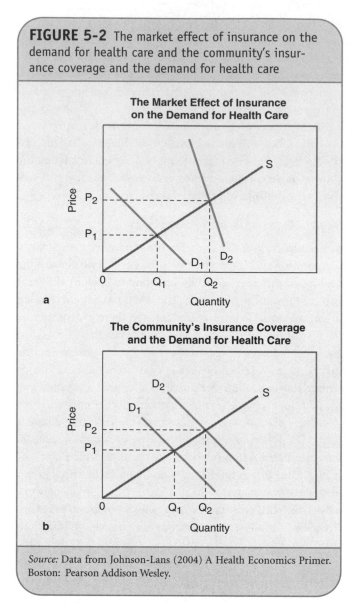

FIGURE 5-2 The market effect of insurance on the demand for health care and the community's insurance coverage and the demand for health care

The Market Effect of Insurance on the Demand for Health Care

The Community's Insurance Coverage and the Demand for Health Care

Source: Data from Johnson-Lans (2004) A Health Economics Primer. Boston: Pearson Addison Wesley.

cent of the increase in healthcare expenditures in the United States between the end of World War II and the mid-1980s was associated with an increase in insurance coverage (Newhouse, 1988).

The majority of economists have agreed that the favorable tax treatment given to health insurance created a welfare loss to society by encouraging workers to purchase more extensive insurance coverage than was socially optimal (Arrow, 1963). The argument was that the tax-free status of employee health insurance led people to be insured to the point where the marginal value of insurance benefits was less than the marginal cost of the insurance in taxable dollars (Feldstein and Friedman, 1977).

The cost to society of subsidizing health insurance was considered to be a function of the price elasticity of demand for health care and the elasticity of supply for healthcare services. The social cost will be greater the lower the elasticity of supply is, because the effect of increased demand for health care will then cause a corresponding increase in price (see Figures 5-2a and b).

A counterargument is that the favorable tax treatment of health insurance, which has also stimulated the growth of employer-based insurance, has increased access to group insurance for those who may not have purchased individual or direct pay insurance. Therefore, the correct measure of welfare loss due to moral hazard would calculate how much extra health care a consumer would demand if he or she purchased an actuarially fair contract when ill (Nyman, 2001). A study by Nyman (2001) addressing the issue of providing health insurance coverage to those previously uninsured found that favorable tax treatment of employer-based insurance would reduce healthcare spending by considerably less than had been predicted in most of the literature, and that more than half of the reduction in spending would result from a decline in the number of people having any coverage, rather than from a reduction in coverage.

INSURANCE TRENDS

Over the past 20 years there has been a noticeable decrease in the amount that employers are willing to pay for insurance premiums. Firms increasingly offer only base-level insurance plans and give employees the option of paying the differences for more extensive coverage if they so choose. Several reasons have been given for this phenomenon in addition to the rise in health insurance premiums—the recession in the late 1980s and early 1990s, the extension of Medicaid coverage to more low-income worker families, and the growth of dual-earner families, which reduced the pressure of employers to cover dependents. The decline in unionizations has been found to explain approximately one quarter of the reduction in the generosity of plans (Buchmueller, 2002). However, the rise in health insurance premiums is a major contributor. In 2002, during the open enrollment period in health insurance plans, premiums quoted were on average 27 percent over the premiums offered in the previous year (Geary, 2002). Similar increases occurred between 2002 and 2003, with at least a 10 percent increase in 2004—which is still two times the inflation rate overall in the United States (Freudenheim, 2004).

Health insurance coverage has declined in large part because workers have not exercised options to purchase it. The rise in insurance premiums and the cutback in the proportion of the premiums that the employers are willing to pay have left many workers without affordable premium costs. Cutler (2002) found a significant drop in take-up rates on the part of employees offered insurance during the period 1998 to 2001. There are important policy implications associated with the fact that a growing proportion of the 44 million uninsured Americans in 2004 were workers and families of employed persons.

SUMMARY

The demand for health insurance exists because of the uncertainty associated with a person's state of health and the risk of very large expenditures in the case of illness. Health insurance provides risk sharing between the insured and insurer, pooling risks among the insured, and sometimes risk sharing between the insurer and healthcare providers. Insurance is a mechanism for transferring funds from the state in which a person is well to the costly state of illness, as well as between people who are well to those requiring health care. Because most private insurance is purchased through the workplace in employer-based plans, there is a degree of community rating involved in the pricing of insurance policies. Group insurance is a mechanism for dealing with adverse selection.

Insurance increases the demand for health care, as well as its price. After decades of discussion, questions still remain about the welfare effects of subsidizing employer-based insurance through favorable tax treatment. Recent literature suggests that there are positive welfare effects associated with increasing access to group insurance, as well as negative effects associated with moral hazard. Increases in premiums and cutbacks in the proportion of the premiums that employers are willing to pay have shifted the focus of policy concerns from whether employees have typical insurance coverage to whether too few have any coverage at all.

Key Words

- Experience rating
- Community rating
- Moral hazard
- Adverse selection
- Managed care organizations
- Private insurance
- Social insurance

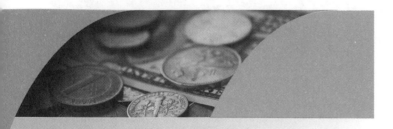

Questions

1. How would you define a risk-neutral person in the context of making decisions about health insurance?

2. What is meant by a loading fee when we consider the price of an insurance policy? Why is the loading fee a higher proportion of the premium when people choose low deductibles?

3. Define moral hazard and provide an example.

4. What are advantages and disadvantages of community rating of health insurance? Consider both equity and efficiency.

REFERENCES

1. Arrow, KJ. (1963) Uncertainty and the welfare economics of medical care. *American Economic Review*, 5:941–972.

2. Buchmueller, T et al. (2002) Union effects on health insurance provision and coverage in the United States. *Industrial and Labor Relations Review*, 55:610–627.

3. Buchmueller, T and J DiNardo. (1999) *Did Community Rating Induce an Adverse Selection Death Spiral? Evidence from New York, Pennsylvania and Connecticut.* NBER Working Paper No. 6872. Cambridge MA: National Bureau of Economic Research.

4. Cutler, DM. (2002) *Employer Costs and the Decline in Health Insurance Coverage.* NBER Working Paper No. W9036. Cambridge, MA: National Bureau of Economic Research.

5. Cutler, DM and RJ Zeckhauser. The anatomy of health insurance. In: Cuyler, AJ and JP Newhouse, eds. *Handbook of Health Economics*, Vol. 1A. Amsterdam: Elsevier; 2000.

6. Feldstein, MS and B Friedman. (1977) Tax subsidies: The rational demand for insurance and the health care crisis. *Journal of Public Economics*, 7:155–178.

7. Freudenheim, M. (2004) Increase in health care premiums are slowing. *New York Times*, May 27: C1.

8. Geary, LH. (2002) Choosing your health plan. *CNN/MONEY.com*, November 1.

9. Gruber, J. Health insurance and the labor market. In: Cuyler, AJ and JP Newhouse, eds. *Handbook of Health Economics*, Vol. 1A. Amsterdam: Elsevier; 2000.

10. Johnson-Lans, S. (2006) *A Health Economics Primer.* Boston: Pearson Addison Wesley.

11. Morris, S, Devlin, N and D Parkin. (2007) *Economic Analysis in Health Care.* West Sussex, England: John Wiley & Sons, Ltd.

12. Mossialos, E, Dixon, A, Figueras, J, and J Kutzin. (2002) *Funding Health Care Options for Europe. Policy Brief No. 4.* London: European Observatory on Health Care Systems.

13. Newhouse, JP. (1988) Has the erosion of the medical market place ended? *Journal of Health Politics, Policy and Law*, 13:263–277.

14. Nyman, JA. (2001) The income transfer effect, the access value of insurance and the RAND Health Insurance Experiment. *Journal of Health Economics*, 20:295–298.

15. Rothschild, M and J Stiglitz. (1976) Equilibrium in competitive insurance markets: an essay on the economics of imperfect information. *Quarterly Journal of Economics*, 90:629–649.

16. Zweifel, P and WG Manning. Moral hazard and consumer incentives in health care. In: Cuyler, AJ and JP Newhouse, eds. *Handbook of Health Economics*, Vol. 1A. Amsterdam: Elsevier; 2000.

BIO: GARY S. BECKER

Gary S. Becker has inspired a revolution in economic thought, extending the boundaries of economic inquiry and ultimately redefining what economists do. Beginning with his dissertation research published in 1957 as "The Economics of Discrimination," Becker's theoretical work has opened to economists the research fields of other social sciences.

In addition to his early work on discrimination, Becker is responsible for ground breaking research on social issues such as fertility and demographics, education, crime and punishment, and marriage and divorce—all aspects of human behavior once considered outside the scope of economics. He is best known for his contribution to a symposium on "Investment in

Human Beings," published in a special issue of the *Journal of Political Economy* in 1962. This work, expanded into a book in 1964 entitled *Human Capital*, is recognized as a classic piece of research by economists and serves as the theoretical foundation for a field of study under the same title. Within this framework, individuals spend and invest in themselves and their children with the future in mind. Education and training, job search, migration, and medical care are all viewed as investments in human capital.

Later research into crime and punishment and the economics of family has been equally revolutionary, affecting not only economics but also criminology and sociology. In 1992, Becker became the third straight University of Chicago economist to be awarded the Nobel Prize for economics for extending "the domain of microeconomic analysis to a wide range of human behavior and interaction including nonmarket behavior."

Becker graduated from Princeton in 1951. He completed his doctoral training at the University of Chicago in 1955 and remained there as part of their faculty. Except for 12 years at Columbia University and the National Bureau of Economic Research, Becker has maintained his Chicago affiliation throughout his professional career. Becker's unrivaled imagination saved economics from irrelevancy.

Source: JR Shackleton. (1981) "Gary S. Becker: The Economist as Empire-Builder." In J.R. Shackleton and G. Locksley, eds. Twelve Contemporary Economists (New York: MacMillan).

Health Economics and Policy, 2nd Edition. James W. Henderson. (Cincinnati, OH: South-western, 2002).

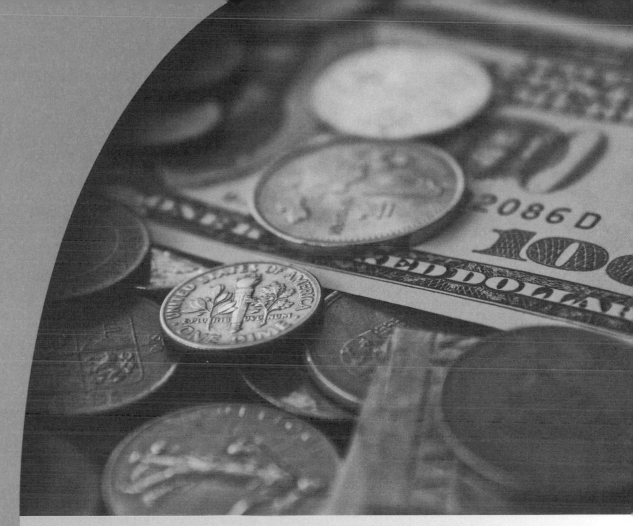

PART III

SUPPLY

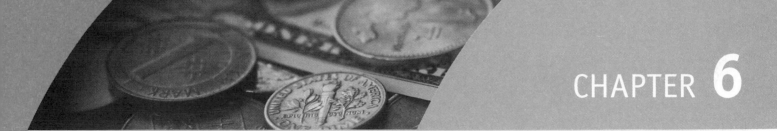

CHAPTER **6**

Healthcare Production, Costs, and Supply

THE NATURE OF PRODUCTION

Because the production and sale of healthcare goods takes place in a world of scarce resources, microeconomics can provide valuable insights into the operation and planning process of medical firms. In this chapter, various economic principles will be used to guide the production and cost behavior of medical firms.

Five assumptions are made to simplify the discussion of short run production: 1) Assume the firm produces a single output of medical services; 2) initially assume that only two inputs exist: personnel hours and a composite capital good; 3) assume that capital is fixed during the period because short run is defined as a period where at least one input is fixed; 4) assume that the firm initially has the incentive to produce as efficiently as possible; and 5) initially assume that the firm possesses perfect information regarding the demands for its product (Santerre and Neun, 2007).

A **production function** identifies how various inputs can be combined and transformed into a final output. The short run production function for healthcare services can be mathematically generalized as $q = f(n, k)$, where q is output, n is personnel hours, and k is capital (which is fixed in the short run).

The production function allows for the possibility that each level of output may be produced by several different combinations of personnel and capital inputs. Each combination is assumed to be technically efficient because it results in the maximum amount of output that is feasible given the state of technology (Johnson-Lans, 2006).

The Healthcare Production Function

The analysis begins by examining the level of healthcare services, q, as it relates to a greater quantity of variable personnel input, n, given that the capital amount, k, is assumed to be fixed. One important microeconomic principle from production theory is the law of diminishing marginal returns. This phenomenon occurs when total output at first increases at an increasing rate, but after some point increases at a decreasing rate with respect to a greater quantity of a variable input, holding all other inputs constant.

Figure 6-1 shows the law of diminishing productivity. It shows a graphical relation between the quantity of healthcare services on the vertical axis and the number of personnel hours on the horizontal axis. The curve is the total product curve, TP, because it depicts the total output produced by different levels of variable input, holding all other inputs constant. The output first increases at an increasing rate over the range of personnel hours of 0 to n_1. Beyond point n_1, further increases in personnel hours cause healthcare services to increase, but at a decreasing rate. That is the point at which diminishing productivity sets in. Beyond n_2, the possibility is that too many personnel hours can lead to a reduction in the quantity of healthcare services. The slope of the total product curve is negative beyond n_2 (Johnson-Lans, 2006).

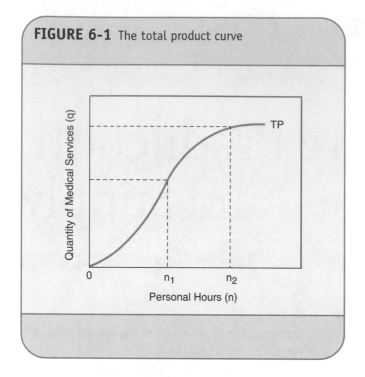

FIGURE 6-1 The total product curve

Economists point to the fixed short run inputs as a basis for diminishing productivity. For example, when personnel hours are increased, at first there is initially a considerable amount of capital, the fixed input, with which to produce healthcare services. The abundance of capital enables increasingly greater amounts of healthcare services to be generated from the employment of additional personnel. At some point, however, the fixed capital becomes limited relative to the variable input, and additional personnel hours lead to successively fewer incremental units of healthcare output. In the extreme case, as more personnel are crowded into a medical facility, the quantity of services produced may begin to decline as congestion sets in and creates unwanted production problems (Johnson-Lans, 2006).

Elasticity of Input Substitution

Realistically, however, the medical firm operates with more than one variable input in the short run. Therefore, there may be some form of substitutability between variable inputs. For example, licensed practical nurses often substitute for registered nurses in the production of inpatient services. The actual degree of substitutability between any two inputs depends on technical and legal considerations. For example, physician assistants are prohibited by law from prescribing medications in most states.

In general terms, the elasticity of substitution between any two variable inputs equals the percent change in input ratio divided by the percent change in the ratio of the inputs' mar-

ginal productivities, holding the level of output constant. In other words, the formula for this elasticity is:

$$\sigma = \frac{\Delta(i_1/i_2)}{i_1/i_2} \div \frac{\Delta(MP_2/MP_1)}{MP_2/MP_1}$$

where i is the quantity employed of each input (Johnson-Lans, 2004). The ratio of marginal productivities is referred to as the marginal rate of technical substitution, which illustrates the rate at which one input substitutes for the other in the production process, at the margin. The marginal product is the additional quantity of output associated with an additional unit of a variable input. For example, suppose two licensed practical nurse hours are needed to substitute completely for one registered nurse hour.

Theoretically, σ takes on the value between 0 and $+ \infty$ and identifies the percent change in the input ratio that results from a 1 percent change in the marginal rate of technical substitution. At the extremes, there is either no substitutability (i.e., 0), or infinite, or perfect substitutability.

SHORT RUN COSTS FOR A MEDICAL FIRM

Economists and accountants refer to costs differently. Accountants considers only the explicit costs of doing business when determining the accounting profits of a medical firm. Explicit costs are easily identified because a recent market transaction is available to provide an accurate measure of costs. Wage payments to staff, utility bills, and medical supply expenses are all examples of explicit costs of healthcare firms (Santerre and Neun, 2007).

Economists consider both the explicit and implicit costs of production. Implicit costs reflect the opportunity costs of using any resources the medical firm owns. For example, a general practitioner (GP) may own the physical assets used in producing physician services. In this case, a recent market transaction is unavailable to determine the cost of using these assets. However, an opportunity cost is incurred when using them because the physical assets could have been rented out for an alternative use. For example, the clinic could be remodeled and rented as a psychological counseling center, and the medical equipment could be rented by another physician. Therefore, the foregone rental payments reflect the opportunity cost of using the physical assets owned by the GP (Johnson-Lans, 2006).

When determining the economic profit of a firm, economists consider the total costs of doing business, including both the explicit and implicit costs. Economists believe it is important to determine whether sufficient revenues are available to cover the costs of using all inputs, including those rented and owned. For example, if the rental return on the physical assets is greater than the return on use, the GP might do better by renting out the assets rather than retaining them for personal use.

Short Run Cost Curve

Cost theory on the production theory of the medical firm previously outlined relates the quantity of output to the cost of production. As such, it identifies how total costs respond to changes in output. If we continue to assume the two inputs of personnel hours, n, and capital, k (still fixed), the short run total costs, STC, of producing a given level of medical output, q, can be written as:

$$STC(q) = wn + r\bar{k}$$

where w and r represent the wage for personnel and the rental or opportunity costs of capital, respectively. Input prices are assumed to be fixed, which means the single medical firm can purchase these inputs without affecting their market prices. This is a valid assumption as long as the firm is a buyer of inputs relative to the total number of buyers in the marketplace (Santerre and Neun, 2007).

The equation above implies that the short run total costs of production are dependent on the quantities and prices of inputs employed. The wage rate times the number of personnel hours equals the total wage bill and represents the total variable costs of production. Variable costs respond to changes in total output. The product of the rental price and the quantity of capital represent the total fixed costs of production. This cost component does not vary with the level of production because the quantity of capital is fixed (Johnson-Lans, 2006).

The total product curve not only identifies the quantity of healthcare output produced by a particular number of personnel hours, but also shows, reciprocally, the number of personnel hours necessary to produce a given level of healthcare output. With this information, the short run total cost can be determined for various levels of healthcare output. First, through the production function, the necessary number of personnel hours , n, for each level of medical output is determined. Second, the quantity of personnel hours are multiplied by the hourly wage to get the short run total variable costs (STVC) of production, or wn. Third, the short run total fixed costs are added, (STFC or rk) to the STVC to derive the short run total costs (STC) of production. This three-step procedure for each level of output can be used to derive the short run total cost curve like the one in Figure 6-2 (Johnson-Lans, 2006).

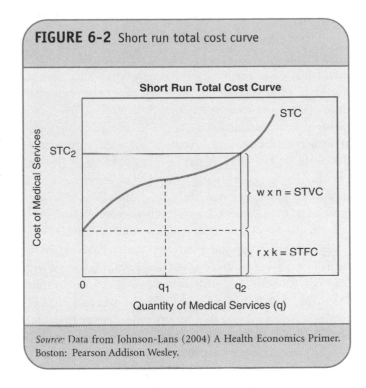

FIGURE 6-2 Short run total cost curve

Source: Data from Johnson-Lans (2004) A Health Economics Primer. Boston: Pearson Addison Wesley.

There is a reciprocal relation between the short run total **cost function** in Figure 6-2 and the short run total product curve in Figure 6-1. For example, when total product is increasing at an increasing rate up to point n_1 in Figure 6-1, short run total costs are increasing at a decreasing rate up to output q_1 in Figure 6-2. In practice, distinguishing between total fixed and total variable costs can be particularly challenging.

Factors Affecting the Position of the Short Run Cost Curve

A variety of short run circumstances affect the position of the total cost curve. Among them are the prices of variable inputs, the quality of care, the patient case-mix, and the amounts of the fixed inputs. Whenever any one of these variables changes, the position of the cost curve changes through either an upward or a downward shift depending on whether costs increase or decrease. A properly specified short run total variable cost function for medical services should include the following variables:

$$STVC = f(\text{output level, input prices, quality of care, patient case-mix, quantity of the fixed inputs})$$
(Johnson-Lans, 2006)

LONG RUN COSTS

Long run **economies of scale** refer to the notion that average costs fall as a medical firm gets physically larger due to specialization of labor and capital. Larger medical firms are able to utilize larger and more specialties in the various labor tasks involved in the production process. For example, people generally get very proficient at a specific task when they perform it repeatedly. Therefore, specialization allows larger firms to produce increased amounts of output at lower costs. The downward sloping portion of the long run average total cost curve (*LATC*) in Figure 6-3 reflects economies of scale.

Another way to conceptualize long run economies of scale is through a direct relation between inputs and output, or returns to scale, rather than output and costs. Consistent with long run economies of scale is **increasing returns** to scale. Increasing returns to scale result when an increase in all inputs results in a more than proportionate increase in output. For example, a doubling of all inputs that result in three times as much output is a sign of increasing returns to scale. Similarly, if a doubling of output can be achieved without doubling of all inputs, the production process exhibits long run increasing returns, or economies of scale.

Most economists believe that economies of scale are exhausted at some point and **diseconomies of scale** set in. Diseconomies of scale result when the medical firm becomes too large. Bureaucratic red tape becomes common, and top-to-bottom communication flows break down. As a result, poor decisions are sometimes made. Consequently, as the firm gets too large, long run average costs increase. Diseconomies of scale are reflected in the upward sloping segment of the *LATC* curve in Figure 6-3.

Diseconomies of scale can also be interpreted to mean that an increase in all inputs results in a less than proportionate increase in output, or **decreasing returns** to scale. For example, if the number of painter hours doubles at a dental office and the decision maker is forced to triple the size of each input (staff, office space, etc.) in order to have some increase in services, the production process at the dental office is characterized by decreasing returns or diseconomies of scale.

Another possibility shown in Figure 6–3 is that the production process exhibits constant returns to scale. Constant returns to scale occur when, for example, a doubling of inputs results in a doubling of output. In terms of long run costs, constant returns imply a horizontal *LATC* curve; in turn implying that long run average costs are independent of output.

Shifts in the Long Run Average Cost Curve

The position of the long run average cost curve is determined by a set of long run circumstances that includes the price of all inputs, quality, and patient case-mix. When these circumstances change on a long run basis, the long run average cost curve shifts up or down depending on whether the change involved higher or lower long run costs of production. For example, a cost-saving technology tends to shift the long run average cost curve down (Johnson-Lans, 2006).

THE NATURE OF SUPPLY

The supply of health care can be approached in a similar way as the demand for health care. Suppliers include hospitals, which provide health care directly, and medical equipment and pharmaceutical companies, which provide inputs to the healthcare production process. The supply side of the market is heavily dependent on theories of how firms behave—this concept is often called the theory of the firm (Morris et al., 2007).

Analysis of supply in economics is often dominated by theories of the firm that are based on an assumption that

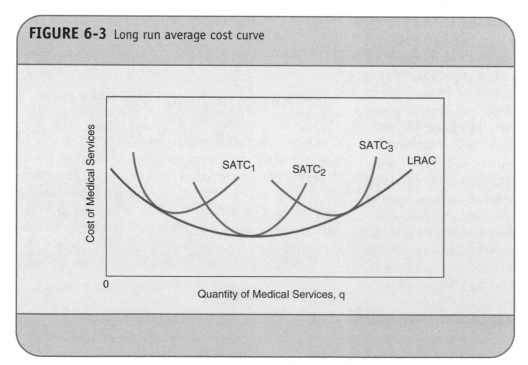

FIGURE 6-3 Long run average cost curve

their overriding aim is to maximize profits. This can be viewed in two ways. First, such theories can be reasonable descriptions of the aims of some firms and can therefore be used in a positive economics sense to generate predictions about the ways that firms and markets operate. However, a typical characteristic of healthcare operations is that not only do firms not aim to maximize profits, but they do not aim to earn any excess profits at all. All firms must earn a normal rate of return or profit if they are going to be able to remain in business in the long run. The aim of most pharmaceutical companies and many insurance companies is to generate profits, and profit maximization may be a reasonable goal for them. By contrast, most hospitals and nursing homes and some insurance companies do not aim to maximize profit. However, theories based on profit maximization have a second use because they provide a useful set of performance benchmarks against which firms' actual performance can be compared. Therefore, even though profit maximization models are important, we will stress that for much of the healthcare industry other theories will be more appropriate (Johnson-Lans, 2006).

Figure 6-4 shows an upward sloping supply curve for office visits. It illustrates, for example, that physicians would be willing to offer ten office visits if the price were $90 per visit. At a higher price, say $100, more visits would be offered.

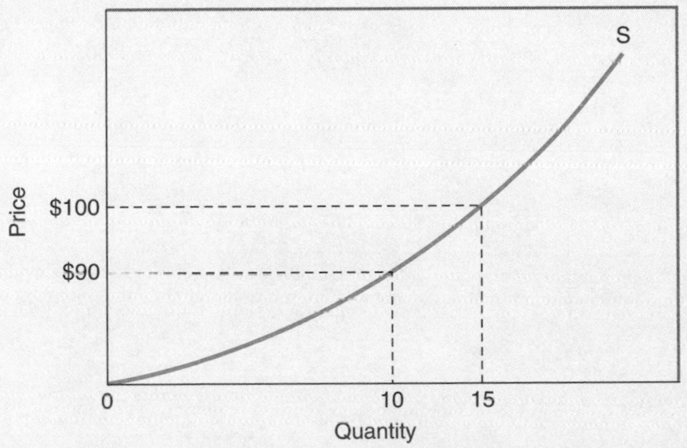

Factors that Affect Supply

We may also generate a list of supply shifters. The following are exogenous determinants of supply; in other words, factors that are held constant underlying the supply curve. The supply curve denotes the relationship between the price of the output and the quantity supplied of the output at the specified prices. Output price is considered an endogenous determinant of supply.

1. *Technological change.* As technology improves for producing a healthcare product, the goods become cheaper to produce. Certainly, technological changes that make products more costly without improving quality are ignored. As the product becomes cheaper to produce, suppliers are willing to offer more for sale at a given price. This increases supply, thus shifting the supply curve to the right.
2. *Input prices.* If the wages of physicians were to rise, this increase in an input cost would result in suppliers' willingness to offer as much for sale at the original price. The supply would decrease, shifting the curve to the left.
3. *Prices of production-related goods.* The price of a good related to production, such as a rise in the price of radiology services, also would be relevant. Because physicians can use radiology for diagnosis as well as treatment, this will cause the supply to decrease, thus shifting the supply curve to the left.
4. *Size of the industry.* As more firms enter the market, the supply of the product will be greater. Therefore, entry of firms will cause the supply curve to shift to the right.
5. *Weather.* For a number of products, acts of God such as weather will tend to affect production. The direction of the effect is obvious: good weather increases supply.

SUMMARY

In this chapter, the characteristics and concepts pertaining to the costs of producing healthcare services were presented. First, the underlying production behavior of a

FIGURE 6-4 Supply of office visits

single medical firm was described. The short run production function that resulted from this examination relates productivity to input usage. Second, the inverse relation between productivity and costs was presented. Finally, some concepts, such as economies of scale and returns to scale, were defined.

In any market, including the market for healthcare services, there is a direct relationship between price and quantity supplied. That is, as price increases, the quantity offered for sale in the market will increase. Several other underlying factors affect the position of the supply curve, shifting it to the left or right as noted previously.

Key Words

- Production function
- Cost function
- Economies of scale
- Increasing returns
- Diseconomies of scale
- Decreasing returns

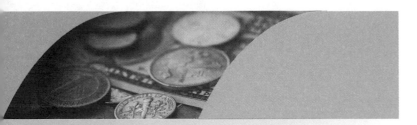

REFERENCES

1. Johnson-Lans, S. (2004) *A Health Economics Primer.* Boston: Pearson Addison Wesley.
2. Johnson-Lans, S. (2006) *A Health Economics Primer.* Boston: Pearson Addison Wesley.
3. Morris S, Devlin, N, and D Parkin. (2007) *Economic Analysis in Health Care.* West Sussex, England: John Wiley & Sons, Ltd.
4. Santerre, RE and SP Neun. (2007) *Health Economics: Theories, Insights and Industry Studies,* 4th ed. Mason, Ohio: Thomson South-Western.

Questions

1. Suppose you are to specify a short run production function for counseling services. What inputs might you include in the production function? Which would be variable inputs and which would be fixed inputs?

2. What does the elasticity of substitution illustrate?

3. Explain the difference between explicit and implicit costs of production.

4. Explain the reasoning behind the U-shaped long run average cost curve.

5. Suppose that licensure requirements become more stringent so that fewer physicians will be able to practice medicine. What would happen to the supply curve for physician services? Explain.

6. Suppose there is a high demand for a new diet drug on the market. What would happen to the supply of the drug?

BIO: RICHARD G. FRANK

Richard G. Frank, PhD, is the Margaret T. Morris Professor of Health Economics in the Department of Health Care Policy at Harvard Medical School. He is also a research associate with the National Bureau of Economic Research. Dr. Frank is engaged in research in three general areas: the economics of mental health care, the economics of the pharmaceutical industry, and the organization and financing of physician group practices.

Dr. Frank and his colleagues are examining competing strategies for organizing and financing mental health and substance abuse care under research grants from the Hogg Foundation, the Robert Wood Johnson Foundation, and the National Institute of Drug Abuse. Under grants from NIDA and the MacArthur Foundation, Dr. Frank and colleagues are studying the performance of social insurance programs for people with mental and addictive disorders. Dr. Frank's work in the area of pharmaceuticals has focused on drug pricing and the dynamics of competition. He has also conducted studies on the impact of prescription drug formularies and the economics of new psychotropic drugs. The third area of activity involves understanding the economic and organizational factors that influence the performance of medical group practices. Dr. Frank and his colleagues are studying the organizational, managerial, and financial factors that explain variation in the performance of medical group practices.

Dr. Frank serves on the Congressional Citizen's Working Group on Health Care. He advises several state mental health and substance abuse agencies on issues related to managed care and financing of care. In 1997, Dr. Frank was elected to the Institute of Medicine. He was awarded the Georgescu-Roegen prize from the Southern Economic Association for work on drug pricing, the Carl A. Taube Award from the American Public Health Association, and the Emily Mumford Medal from Columbia University's Department of Psychiatry. In 2002, Dr. Frank received the John Eisberg Mentorship Award from National Research Service Awards. He received a BA in economics from Bard College and a PhD in economics from Boston University.

Source: Richard G. Frank curriculum vita. Harvard University Web site.

The Healthcare Workforce Market

THE MARKET FOR PHYSICIANS AND NURSES

Two differing points of view have characterized American attitudes toward medical professionals in the United States. One focuses on the high monetary and psychological costs of the lengthy training period, long hours, and great responsibility that being a practicing physicians entails and concludes that the economic returns to practicing medicine are not excessive. The other viewpoint asserts that physicians and other healthcare providers have been able to extract economic rents by charging fees that are higher than those which prevail in a reasonably competitive market (Nova Online, 2001).

This chapter will focus on the supply of physicians and nurses and, in particular, their decisions to undertake training and enter the field of medicine. Health planners define the adequacy of the supply of doctors and nurses in relation to the community's health needs. Economists use supply and demand to analyze the markets for doctors and nurses. This analysis is applied to understanding why shortages and surpluses may exist.

THE PHYSICIAN'S MARKET

The supply of physicians depends upon a combination of individual career decisions and public policy. Since the middle of

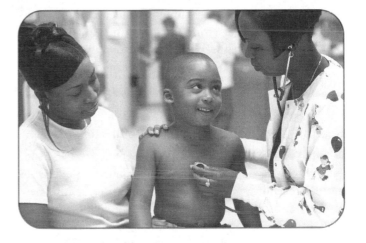

the nineteenth century, medical associations have interacted with state and federal governments to regulate the practice of medicine. Medical schools and hospitals with residency programs also make decisions that affect the opportunities for training. As a result, individuals' ability to enter the profession and the financial returns of doing so are not left to the invisible hand of the supply and demand in the private market (Johnson-Lans, 2006).

The professionalization of medical training and the practice of medicine date from the mid-nineteenth century, when at the urging of the **American Medical Association (AMA)**, state licensing boards were established to set examinations for doctors of medicine (MDs). Licensing limited the scope of activity of other medical practitioners: homeopaths, osteopaths, chiropractors, midwives, etc. In the twentieth century, the AMA also began to oversee the quality of medical education. In 1910, a commissioned study that came to be known as the Flexner Report. This highly critical review of the medical education led to the closure of many United States medical schools and the addition of a second requirement for becoming a licensed physician graduating from an accredited medical school (Kessel, 1958). The MD degree requires four years of medical school, plus a year-long internship of practical training in hospitals. Physicians must pass examinations in a particular state in order to be licensed to practice there. Most physicians in the United States also undertake additional postgraduate training in the form of hospital residency in some specialty. This is now often combined with the internship. In addition, many become board-certified specialists. A board-certified specialist must complete one or more residencies and pass an examination in one of two specialist fields chosen. A physician can practice in a specialist field, such as cardiology, without being board certified, but the certification carries with it prestige and the likelihood of higher earnings. Some specialists, such as neurosurgeons, require very long residencies. A physician's training often requires a commitment of more than a decade. In 2001, approximately 67 percent of the total actively practicing physicians in the United States were board certified specialists (Pasko and Smart, 2003).

PHYSICIAN SHORTAGE?

Health Planners' Evaluation of the Physician Supply

Health planners evaluate the supply of physicians by looking at the theoretical number of physicians required to perform the health procedures needed by a community, estimating need by referring to statistics on incidence of disease in a population of a given size. Using this definition, it was determined that there was a physician shortage, particularly in certain regions in the early 1960s, given the uneven geographical distribution of practicing physicians (Rimlinger and Steele, 1968).

Economic Analysis of Physician Supply

Economists define a shortage as a situation in which quantity supplied is less than quantity demanded at a given market price. Shortages are not easy to measure in a profession where a high proportion of the members are self-employed. Except for young physicians in training employed by hospitals, there are few data on vacancy rates. Researchers studying markets for professionals therefore study relative earnings or relative returns to training.

Higher earnings in one professional field such as physicians' services, do not necessarily indicate barriers to entry into that field. Earnings differences may simply reflect "compensating differentials" for differences in length and cost of training. The returns to training is a useful measure for analyzing indi-vidual decisions to enter healthcare training and the choices about which field within medicine to pursue (Becker, 1963). Incorporating the human capital model into the analysis of the supply of physicians led to an approach that focused on returns over the lifetime of training rather than current earnings.

A medical degree can be thought of as a stock of human capital that yields a stream of returns over time. A convenient way to evaluate the return on any form of investment is to find its discounted present value (*DPV*), where:

$$DPV = \Sigma[R_{t=} + R_{t+}/(1 + r) + \ldots + R_{t+n}/(1 + r)^{t + n - 1})]$$

The internal rate of return is defined as the discount rate that will equate the (discounted) present value of the return streams with the (discounted) present value of the training costs. Internal rates of return in different professions would be expected to converge over time in competitive markets with freedom of entry. Higher rates of return may be an indication of what are considered to be dynamic shortages. These occur when there are lags in adjustment between supply and demand. In a career where training can take over ten years, the lags can be lengthy and there can be miscalculations about the economic return on the part of those entering the field, especially because supply and demand conditions may shift during the training period. However, because people are attracted to fields with higher returns, persistent differentials in internal rates of return provide indirect evidence of market imperfections (Johnson-Lans, 2004).

In the 1950s and 1960s, physicians were found to receive higher internal rates of return on their training compared with the other professions (Lee et al., 1964). Therefore, economists and health planners concurred that there was a shortage of physicians.

Barriers to Entry

One reason for the higher returns to medical training is that it is a result of **barriers to entry** to practicing medicine. The limited number of places in United States medical schools and the licensing requirements, coupled with immigration policy, greatly restricted the entry of foreign-trained physicians, which could explain the higher than equilibrium returns to medical training. Some economists linked the high returns to profit maximizing behavior on the part of the AMA (Friedman and Kuznets, 1945). The AMA was viewed as a guild that imposed strict apprenticeship requirements and limited entry to the profession. If demand remains constant, imposing restrictions on the number of physicians will increase the price of their services, even if the reason for the restriction is quality control. Also, if entry restrictions are coupled with rules prohibiting price competition, monopoly level prices could result, even when there are many suppliers of the same service (Kessel, 1958). County medical associations had the power to impose sanctions on physicians if they did not cooperate, so the lack of price competition was not an unreasonable assumption. The sanctions could include loss of hospital privileges and exclusion from the medical association, among other things.

In a competitive market with freedom of entry, the equilibrium price for a service would be PC and the equilibrium quantity would be qC. Restrictions on supply are shown in Figure 7-1 as a movement from SS to S_1S_1, with a resulting competitive price of P^*. If physicians' associations set prices collusively within local areas, the profit-maximizing price will approach P_m in the figure (Johnson-Lans, 2006).

Policy Responses to a Shortage

Public policy in the 1960s had the goal of relieving the doctor shortage. The Immigration Act of 1965 made it easier for internationally trained physicians to practice medicine in the United States. The Health Professions Education Act of 1965 increased federal assistance to medical schools, but required them to increase enrollments in order to qualify (Johnson-Lans, 2004). These measures led to an approximate doubling in the size of physician training programs and a significant increase in the number of physicians between 1965 and 1980 (Barzanski, 1991).

By 1970, returns to physicians training, adjusted for hours worked, had become approximately equal to the returns to lawyers and dentists, but were still higher than the returns to other professions requiring graduate degrees (Mennemeyer, 1978). By 1991, internal rates of return to physicians were comparable to, and in the case of primary care physicians, lower than the returns to training to business or law (Johnson-Lans, 2006).

Choice of Specialization

Physicians are not a homogeneous group. Very few physicians in the United States today have only the basic MD degree. Primary care physicians usually complete residencies in fields such as internal medicine or geriatrics.

The proportion of graduates of United States medical schools undertaking residencies in internal medicine declined by over 30 percent between 1986 and 1994. This means that an ever higher proportion of physicians in the primary care field had their training outside of the United States. There was a decline of 45 percent over the same time period in office-based primary care physicians in urban settings (Bindman, 1994). Higher earnings, greater prestige, and also more regular hours attracted physicians to other specialties (McKay, 1990). However, between 1996 and 2001 the proportion of physicians in the practice of primary care was stabilized and remained roughly constant.

Economic Incentives to Alter the Distribution of Physicians

Subsidies for medical training in the form of below-market and deferred interest bearing loans to students and subsidies to medical schools and teaching hospitals for residency training programs result in private costs of training that are much lower than the total costs to society (or social costs). Individuals' decisions about how much training to undertake are based on private costs and returns. Individuals will undertake additional training until the private marginal return on an additional unit of training is just equal to the private marginal

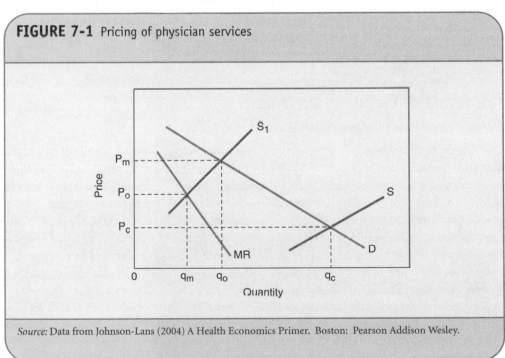

FIGURE 7-1 Pricing of physician services

Source: Data from Johnson-Lans (2004) A Health Economics Primer. Boston: Pearson Addison Wesley.

costs. This may result in a less than ideal distribution of specialists from society's point of view.

Optimality, from the societal viewpoint, is achieved when the marginal social benefit is just equal to the marginal social cost of the last unit of a good or service produced. If there is a divergence between society's goals and the incentives provided by the private market, society's goals are not likely to be achieved unless the incentive structure is changed (Johnson-Lans, 2006).

Public Policy to Change Incentives

The United States government has a policy of forgiving a limited number of student loans for physicians who agree to practice medicine in underserved geographical areas under the National Health Service Corps (Cullen et al., 1994). Changes in the fee structure of Medicare to favor primary care physicians can also be viewed as a public policy designed to alter the supply of physicians in different specialties.

Private Insurance Market Incentives

The enhanced use of primary care physicians in managed care organizations increases the opportunity for primary care physicians. Increased market penetration by managed care insurers during the period 1985 to 1993 was found to be associated with a narrowing of the difference between earnings of primary care physicians and specialists such as radiologists, anesthesiologists, and pathologists (Simon et al., 1998). Metropolitan areas with greater managed care organization penetration experienced slower rates of growth in specialists and in total number of physicians, but no change in the rate of growth in general practitioners, during the period of 1987 to 1997 (Escarce et al., 2000).

THE RESULT OF CHANGING INCENTIVES

Fields Chosen by Younger Physicians

The distribution of physicians by specialty shows a different pattern if we take account of age. By 2001, over half of the female and over 40 percent of the male physicians under the age of 35 were practicing in the fields of internal medicine, family practice, and pediatrics (American Medical Association, 1998). Physicians under the age of 35 in 2001 who were trained in the United States would have been making decisions about specialty fields beginning in approximately 1991, when Medicare payment reforms were already in place and managed care was making serious inroads into national markets. Other factors also influenced the specialty decisions, including guaranteed vacations, more certain work schedules, and shorter periods of residency training (Thornton and Esposito, 2003).

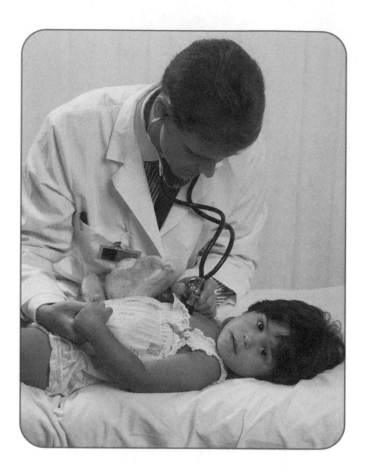

PROJECTIONS ABOUT THE SUPPLY AND DEMAND OF PHYSICIANS: ECONOMIC AND HEALTH PLANNING VIEWPOINTS

By the late 1970s, it was widely believed that there had been a policy overshoot and an oversupply of physicians would soon develop. Congress, concerned whether Medicare would continue to provide several billion dollars per year in support of residency programs, established the Council on Graduate Medical Education. This concluded that, by the year 2000, the overall physician to population ratio would be high. It also predicted that the specialists would be 60 percent higher than needed. It recommended that subsidies to hospital residency programs be reduced, and more medical students be directed to the field of primary care (Weiner, 2003). The number of openings in United States medical schools was stabilized and remained rather constant.

Predictions about the future supply of physicians vary. Some see a shortage looming ahead, but this view is not universally accepted. In 2001, a roundtable discussion provided a representative sample of views on this issue. The difference between the economists' view and the health planners' opinions is revealed in this representative sample of expert opinions.

THE MARKET FOR NURSES

Nurses will be referred in this chapter to mean registered nurses (RNs). There are three different paths to achieving an RN degree. Two-year associate programs in community colleges and three-year diploma programs in hospitals coexist with BA programs in four-year colleges. Graduate programs in nursing, leading to an MA or PhD are also available. Registered nurses, like physicians, can get additional training in specialist areas. As the production function for healthcare changes, the demand for nurses is affected (Johnson-Lans, 2004).

The main employer of registered nurses has traditionally been the hospital, even though by the end of the 1990s the proportion of nurses employed in hospitals had fallen to about 60 percent (Feldstein, 1999). The greater intensity of care within acute care hospitals increases the desired nurse-to-patient ratio and the demand for hospital nurses, but a reduction in the use of inpatient hospital services tends to reduce nurse employment in hospitals. To the extent that managed

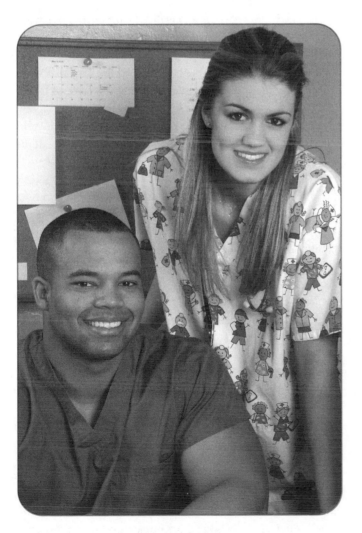

care organizations and other integrated healthcare delivery systems are able to substitute nurses for physicians in ambulatory settings, this tends to increase the demand for nurses in nonhospital settings.

The supply of nurses depends on the decisions of individuals to undertake training and to work in the nursing profession once training is completed. Public policy is just as important in determining the training opportunities for nurses as it is for physicians. The relative rate of return to this occupation compared to other occupations that require comparable training undoubtedly affects the supply. Opportunities for women to become physicians undoubtedly provide an alternative for those who might otherwise enter the nursing profession. As the proportion of male RNs has remained under 5 percent, we cannot assume that a substitution of male for female nurses will do much to offset the increase in other professional opportunities for women (Johnson-Lans, 2004).

IS THERE A NURSING SHORTAGE?

There have been many allegations of a nursing shortage, using both the healthcare planners' and economists' definitions of shortages. The American Hospital Association complained of a nursing shortage in the 1950s and 1960s and supported these claims by noting the high vacancy rates in registered nurse positions and the substitution of less highly trained licensed practical nurses for RNs. The demand for nurses was greater than the supply at the going wage rate. From the 1940s to the early 1960s, vacancy rates for hospital nurses never fell below 13 percent and reached a level of 23 percent in 1962 (Yett, 1975).

Congress responded by passing the Nurse Training Act (NTA) in 1964, which began a tradition of government subsidization of nurses' training. Using vacancy rates in hospitals as an indicator, the legislation that supported nurses' training appears to have mitigated the shortages. Vacancy rates fell to below 10 percent by 1971 (Feldstein, 1999).

Between 1971 and the present, there appears to have been a number of periods of adjustment in which high vacancy rates were followed by policy to expand nurses' training, followed by reductions in shortages. Wages have responded, for the most part, to shortages. Because the training period is so much shorter, responses to imbalances in supply and demand are more rapid than in the case of physician training (Johnson-Lans, 2004).

Cyclical Shortages and Responses

Nurses' decisions about whether to enter the labor force and how many hours to work are very cyclical. The reason for this is that a very high proportion of nurses is married and part of two-earner families. They go in and out of the labor force as employment opportunities and real wages change, but also in response to the employment situation of their spouses. Vacancy rates in nursing are typically much lower in periods of economic recession (Johnson-Lans, 2004).

A recession in the early 1980s increased the labor force participation of trained nurses and reduced the vacancy rate to a record low of fewer than 5 percent. However, by the end of the 1980s, it exceeded 12 percent. A decline in the participation rate of nurses when the economy improved, an increase in the demand for hospital nurses, and a decline in entrants into nurses' training in the early 1980s, all contributed to the reemergence of a shortage (Feldstein, 1999). This led to the passage of the Nurse Shortage Reduction Act of 1988, which provided additional subsidies for nurses' training and the Nurse Relief Act of 1989, which relaxed restrictions on the immigration of foreign-trained nurses. The result was a rapid increase in the supply of nurses. Vacancy rates declined again by the mid 1990s due in part to the 1992 recession that was again accompanied by higher participation rates of nurses. However, since then vacancy rates have been rising again in many parts of the nation (Scanlon, 2001).

Wages

From the 1940s to the early 1960s, nurses' wages declined relative to other female professionals despite high vacancy rates. During that same period, nurses who were employed in non-hospital jobs experienced relative increases in wages compared with those employed in the hospital sector (Feldstein, 1999).

The situation changed with the institution of Medicare in 1965. Hospital nurses salaries increased relative to their non-hospital colleagues, and they achieved parity with earnings in other female dominated occupations requiring the same level of education. Price controls in the 1970s restrained nurses' wages, but they rose again as soon as the controls were removed in 1974. Wage levels were maintained throughout the 1980s (Schumacher, 2001). Nurses' real wages increased between 1983 and 1993, followed by a temporary decline from 1993 to 1997 (Schumacher, 2002). The increase in the supply of nurses resulting from the Nurse Shortage Reduction Act of 1988 was probably a factor because vacancy rates also declined during the same period. However, demand-side pressures may also have contributed. Cost-containment policies of managed care insurers have frequently been alleged to result in hospitals skimping on nursing care (Spetz, 1999). However, managed care organizations' penetration in markets appear to have explained at most a very small proportion of the short term real wage decline for nurses in the 1990s (Schumacher, 2001). Since 1998, the wages of hospital nurses have increased both absolutely and relative to wages for other women with comparable education levels (Hirsch and Schumacher, 2004).

THE MONOPSONISTIC MARKET FOR NURSES

Two dominant beliefs about the market for nurses have been the alleged chronic shortage of registered nurses and the sense that nurses are underpaid. The linking of shortages and low wages is counterintuitive. Because a shortage occurs when the quantity demanded is greater than the quantity supplied at a given wage, in a well-functioning competitive market a shortage should be resolved by wages increasing until equilibrium has been restored. The model of **monopsony** has often been used to explain this phenomenon. A monopsonist is a monopoly buyer of nurses, or employer. The market for registered nurses has been used as a classic textbook example of monopsony. If there is only one hospital in the region, it has potential monopsony power over its nursing supply. Several hospitals might collude with respect to wages offered to nurses, in which case the effect would be the same (Johnson-Lans, 2004).

For monopsony to affect market outcomes, the supply curve of workers must be upward sloping, which means that in order to attract more workers, the employer has to raise wages. The supply curve is an average factor costs curve from the point of view of the employer, if we assume that all persons who do the same work are paid an equivalent wage. If a firm is the only firm employing a given kind of worker, it is a wage setter. Therefore, it must look at the marginal costs of hiring additional workers. When the supply curve is upward sloping, the marginal factor cost curve rises more steeply as shown in Figure 7-2. If the firm has to offer a higher wage to get additional workers, it must also raise the wages of workers it already employs (Johnson-Lans, 2004).

The demand schedule for any input into production is its marginal revenue product curve. The demand curve shows the maximum amount that an employer will pay for any given quantity of workers hired. A hospital will not pay more for an extra nurse than the marginal contributions to revenue. A firm will hire workers up to the quantity where the marginal factor cost (MFC) of the last worker just equals the **marginal revenue product** (MRP) of the last worker. This satisfies the profit-maximizing criterion $MR = MC$. In Figure 7-2, (Wg, ND) shows the quantity of nursing help that will be employed and the wage that will be paid by the monopsonist. At ($Wg1$, ND_1), quantity demanded exceeds quantity supplied by ND_1–NS_1. This difference measures the amount of the vacancy. The monopsony model can explain the coexistence of high vacancy rates and lower than competitive wages of nurses (Johnson-Lans, 2004).

The period from the 1940s to the mid 1960s appears to be one in which the monopsony model fits reasonably well. However, this model is less useful in explaining the trends in employment and earnings for registered nurses in the Medicare period. After 1965, real wages for nurses increased along with

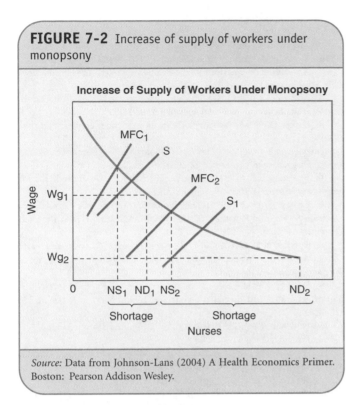

FIGURE 7-2 Increase of supply of workers under monopsony

Increase of Supply of Workers Under Monopsony

Source: Data from Johnson-Lans (2004) A Health Economics Primer. Boston: Pearson Addison Wesley.

demand. The decline in nurses' wages from 1993 to 1997 can be explained without reference to monopsony, but as a result of a rapid increase in supply and some downward pressure in demand for hospital nurses (Johnson-Lans, 2004).

However, economists have revisited the issue of monopsony in the market for nurses. Hospitals have been found to be wage setters and the short run supply of nurses is extremely wage-inelastic (Staiger et al., 1999). Nurses are made to exert more effort when employers have greater market power (Currie et al., 2003). A study of Australian nursing markets makes a strong case for the existence of monopsony there. Australian nurses are paid about 20 percent less than other comparable workers in a period of high vacancy rates (Howak and Preston, 2001). Where monopsony exists, policies to eradicate shortages by increasing the supply of workers may actually increase shortages (Lane and Gohmann, 1995). The American Nurses Association has noted the negative impact of the nurse shortage, which leads to excessive hours of work and rotations to services for which training and experience are inadequate (Spetz, 2002).

A United States government projection of the future supply and demand conditions for RNs shows quantity demanded exceeding quantity supplied by the year 2010. This assumes that nurses' wages are maintained at a constant real level, in other words they are adjusted by expected increases in the price index (Johnson-Lans, 2004).

An innovative way to deal with the hospital nurse shortage is the use of contract labor. Agencies supply nurses on a short-term basis. When nurses supply their labor through these agencies, they sacrifice fringe benefits and job security for higher wages and more flexible hours (Bellemore, 1998). In a profession dominated by married women, this tradeoff may be superior to both the employer and employee. The use of RN temps may be efficient for hospitals facing highly variable demand for nurses. Also, because salaried nurses' wages are not directly affected by the wages paid to temporary workers, employment of nurses might be expanded more than otherwise expected where hospitals have monopsony power (Johnson-Lans, 2004).

SUMMARY

The physician market was historically characterized by barriers to entry leading to higher than competitive rates of return. In the past 15 years, average-hours-adjusted rates of return have been no higher for physicians relative to a variety of other professionals and lower for primary care physicians. Managed care and Medicare appear to have exerted downward pressure on physicians' earnings and have also changed the relative returns to different specialties. This, plus the large increase in the proportion of women physicians, appears to be resulting in a trend toward more primary care physicians. However, as their earnings have increased, they have cut back on the number of hours worked. This results in a relatively smaller increase in primary care physician services. Over time, the view has vacillated between perceived physician shortages and projected surpluses, but overall there has been a persistent geographical maldistribution of physicians.

The historical market for nurses appears to have been one in which the employer had monopoly power. This is the usual explanation for the combination of low wages and high vacancy rates that prevailed from the 1940s to the 1960s. The present situation is that vacancy rates are high, as are wage rates. Projections are that the demand for nurses will outstrip the supply in the next two decades. Some researchers still find evidence of monopsony power. If monopsony is important, increasing the supply of nurses will not be effective in eliminating shortages and may even lead to a larger gap between supply and demand. In that situation, unionization, a minimum nursing wage, or possible a direct wage subsidy to nurses, might help to eliminate the shortages.

Key Words

- AMA
- Barriers to entry
- Monopsony
- Marginal revenue product

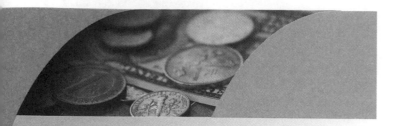

Questions

1. What are the economic reasons for the high ratio of specialists to general practitioners in the United States compared to other countries?

2. The American Medical Association (AMA) has often been thought to behave like a trade union in restricting the supply of physicians in order to keep earnings high. What evidence is there that the AMA has acted this way?

3. Is there a chronic shortage of nurses in the United States? Explain this from both an economist's and health planner's perspectives.

4. The market for nurses has characteristics of monopsony. Outline arguments on both sides of this statement.

REFERENCES

1. American Medical Association, Center for Health Policy Research. (1998) *Physician Marketplace Characteristics, 1997–1998.* Chicago: AMA.

2. Association of American Medical Colleges. (2002) *AAMC Data Book 2002.* Washington, DC: AAMC.

3. Barzanski, B et al. (1991) Education programs in U.S. medical schools. *Journal of the American Medical Association,* 266:916.

4. Becker, G. (1965) A theory of allocation of time. *Economic Journal,* 75:493–517.

5. Bellemore, FA. (1998) Temporary employment decisions of registered nurses. *Eastern Economic Journal,* 24:265–279.

6. Bindman, AB. (1994) Primary and managed care: ingredients for health care reform. *Western Journal of Medicine,* 161:78–82.

7. Cullen, TJ et al. (1994) *The National Health Service Corps: Rural Physician Service and Retention.* Seattle, WA: WAMI Rural Health Research Center.

8. Currie, J et al. (2003) *Cut to the Bone? Hospital Takeovers and Nurse Employment.* NBER Working Paper No. 9428. Cambridge, MA: National Bureau of Economic Research.

9. Escarce, JE et al. (2000) HMO growth and geographical redistribution of generalist and specialist physicians. *Health Services Research,* 35: 825–848.

10. Feldstein, PJ. (1999) *Health Care Economics,* 5th ed. Albany, NY: Delmar Publishers.

11. Friedman, M and S Kuznets. (1945) *Income from Professional Practice.* New York: National Bureau of Economic Research.

12. Hirsch, BT and EJ Schumacher. (2004) *Classic Monopsony or New Monopsony? Searching for Evidence in Nursing Labor Markets,* IZA Discussion paper No. 1154. Chicago: Institute for the Study of Labor.

13. Howak, MJ and AC Preston. (2001) Can human capital theory explain why nurses are so poorly paid? *Australian Economic Papers,* 40:232–245.

14. Johnson-Lans, S. (2006) *A Health Economics Primer.* Boston: Pearson Addison Wesley.

15. Kessel, RA. (1958) Price discrimination in medicine. *Journal of Law and Economics,* 1:20–53.

16. Lane, J and S Gohmann. (1995) Surplus or shortage: economic approaches to the analysis of nursing labor markets. *Southern Economic Journal,* 61:644–653.

17. Lee, B et al. (1968) Migration, location, and remuneration of medical personnel: physicians and dentists. *Review of Economics and Statistics,* 50: 332–347.

18. McKay, NL. (1990) The economic determinants of specialty choice by medical residents. *Journal of Health Care Economics,* 9:335–357.

19. Mennemeyer, ST. (1978) Really great returns to medical education? *Journal of Human Resources,* 13:75–90.

20. Nova Online, (2001) *Survivor M.D., The Hippocratic Oath. Doctor's Responses Set 2.* http://www.pbs.org/wgbh/nova/doctors/oath_modern.html. Accessed March 2005.

21. Pasko, T and DR Smart. (2003) *Physician Characteristics and Distribution in the U.S.* 2003–2004 Edition. Chicago: American Medical Association.

22. Rimlinger, GV and HB Steele. (1968) An economic interpretation of the spatial distribution of physicians in the U.S. *Southern Economic Journal,* 30:1–12.

23. Scanlon, W, (2001) *Nursing Workforce: Recruitment and Retention of Nurses and Nurses Aides Is a Growing Concern.* Washington, DC: U.S. Government Accounting Office.

24. Schumacher, EJ, (2001) The earnings and employment of nurses in an era of cost containment. *Industrial and Labor Relations Review,* 55:116–132.

25. _____ (2002) Technology, skills and health care labor markets. *Journal of Labor Research,* 23:397–415.

26. Simon, CJ et al. (1998) The effect of managed care on the incomes of primary care and specialty physicians. *Health Services Research,* 33:549–569.

27. Spetz, J. (1999) The effects of managed care and prospective payment on the demand for hospital nurses. *Health Services Research*, 34:993–1010.

28. _____ (2002) The value of education in a licensed profession: the choice of associate or baccalaureate degrees in nursing. *Economics of Education Review*, 21:73–85.

29. Staiger, D et al. (1999) *Is There Monopsony in the Labor Market? Evidence from a Natural Experiment*. NBER Working Paper No. 7258. Cambridge, MA: National Bureau of Economic Research.

30 Thornton, J and F Esposito. (2003) How important are economic factors in choice of medical specialty? *Health Economics,* 12:67–73.

31. Weiner, JP. (2003) Perspective: a shortage of physicians or a surplus of assumptions? http://content.Healthaffairs.org/cgi/reprint/21/1/160. Accessed March 2005.

32. Yett, DE. (1975) *An Economic Analysis of the Nurse Shortage*. Lexington, MA: Health.

BIO: THOMAS RICE

Thomas Rice is Professor of the Department of Health Services at the University of California at Los Angeles. He also serves as Vice Chancellor, Academic Personnel for the UCLA campus. He teaches courses in health economics, research methodology, and current issues in health policy.

Dr. Rice received his PhD in Economics at the University of California at Berkeley. He has conducted research projects and published in a number of areas, including: physicians' economic behavior; health insurance for the elderly; the Medicare program; healthcare cost containment; the role of competition in healthcare reform; and managed care.

Dr. Rice has testified before the U.S. Congress numerous times on various health policy issues. In 1988, he received the Association for Health Services Research Young Investigator Award, given to the outstanding health services researcher in the United States age 35 or younger. In 1992, he received the Thompson Prize from the Association for University Programs in Health Administration, awarded annually to the outstanding health services researcher in the country age 40 or under. He was elected to the Institute of Medicine, National Academy of Science, in 2006. In 1998, he received the Article-of-the-Year Award from the Association for Health Services Research. Dr. Rice served as Editor of the journal, *Medical Care Research and Review* from 1994–2000. The second edition of his book, *The Economics of Health Reconsidered*, was published in 2003.

Source: University of California Web site.

Technology Transfer in Health Care

LEARNING OBJECTIVES:

In this chapter, you will learn about:

1. the role of the technology in the production of healthcare services.
2. the process of technological innovation.
3. the efficiency of technological innovations.

TECHNOLOGY IN HEALTH CARE

Health economists and policy analysts are particularly interested in the role of technological change in health care because of the need to assess both its benefits and its impact on the rising costs of health care. A related concern is that cost containment may impede the rate of technological change and its diffusion.

Advances in health care in the second half of the twentieth century raised expectations about attainable levels of health and therefore increased the demand for technologically sophisticated health care. The demand for health care was augmented by the characteristics of the United States health insurance system, which from the 1940s and 1950s imposed no cost controls. The increase in the efficacy of health care and the resulting increase in the cost of health care further augmented the demand for health insurance. Concern over potential medical malpractice lawsuits provided an additional incentive to use the highest technology available. Throughout much of the second half of the twentieth century, the combination of these factors provided a virtual guarantee that the demand for any new innovation could be shown to provide any marginal improvement in treatment outcomes (Johnson-Lans, 2004).

The consensus of those who have worked to identify factors contributing to the increase in the cost of health care is that technology has been the largest contributor to the upward trend in healthcare prices. Considerably less than half of the increase over time in the price of health care can be explained by the combination of increased insurance coverage, increasing real income, supplier-induced demand, monopoly profits to suppliers, changing demographic characteristics of the population, or the labor-intensive character of health care (Newhouse, 1992).

TECHNOLOGICAL CHANGE
Promotion of Innovation

Technological advances take place through the process of innovation. Innovation, which may be integrated with the process of discovery or invention, includes developing and marketing new products. Schumpeter viewed innovation as the driving force in a market economy. He called the process by which one product or process is replaced by a better one "creative destruction." He emphasized the role of profits in stimulating innovation and noted that innovation will be undertaken primarily by firms that have a good deal of market power, such as those that are oligopolies or monopolistically competitive (Schumpeter, 1942). Such factors as professional prestige and the satisfaction derived from helping cure diseases may also be important stimuli in the process of innovation, as is government funding to support basic research.

In the United States, health research takes place within the government-funded National Institutes of Health (NIH); in universities, where much research is also funded by NIH; the National Science Foundation (NSF); and private industry in general and within firms themselves. Studies show that the rate of product development is greater in firms that have more contact with academic institutions, which is particularly true with products that are radically new, rather than incrementally changed products (MacPherson, 2002).

Demand for products and the expectation of profits are needed for innovation to occur. Although government support for research is very important in stimulating innovation, it may not lead to a direct pipeline for commercial products. For instance, a great deal of biotechnology research originating at Oxford and Cambridge Universities has resulted in commercially valuable products being developed in companies outside of the United Kingdom. Price controls on pharmaceuticals imposed by the National Health Service may have contributed to this. There is constant concern in the United States that cost-containment policies have a dampening effect on the rate of innovation in health technology (Baker and Spetz, 1999). The inclusion of price controls on pharmaceutical products may have contributed to the failure of the Clinton health-care reform plan in the 1990s.

Intellectual Property Rights

Another factor that is believed to promote innovation is patent protection for **intellectual property rights**. Patents are permits that grant exclusive ownership rights over processes or products for a specified length of time. In the United States, patents for drugs and medical devices are now granted for a 20-year period, including the testing period. The lengthy testing period often reduces the effective patent life to ten years or less. It is also possible to receive patent protection for new information on individual genes. Patents on biomedical and pharmaceutical innovations may be renewed for up to five years if the Food and Drug Administration (FDA) has delayed the introduction of the new drug onto the market by that long of a period. However, the extension may not be granted for an effective patent life of more than 14 years (Johnson-Lans, 2004).

Without patent protection, innovations would be greatly slowed unless governments were to fund product development, as well as basic research processes. The incentive to innovate would be reduced because duplication makes research and development (R&D) activity less profitable. The problem of imitation is particularly serious in the pharmaceutical industry where development costs are very large compared to production costs. The cost of producing the drugs is minimal compared to the extensive testing to gain governmental approval to market and sell them (Johnson-Lans, 2004).

The relationship between degree of patent protection and the rate of innovation is complicated. This is illustrated by looking at differences across countries. Switzerland, which has been the location of three lucrative pharmaceutical companies, introduced patent protection for drugs only in 1977. Canada had very lax patent laws until 1987, but since strengthening its patent protection, it has experienced a significant increase in R&D activity by attracting foreign multinational firms' research activity (McRae and Tapon, 1985).

U.S. Firms' Successful Innovation

The United States has been the world leader in the commercialization of biotechnical knowledge, although Germany, the United Kingdom, and Canada appear to be beginning to close the gap (Cooke, 2001). The main reasons for the United States' success appear to be:

1. the existence of a large stock of human capital and research institutions
2. government support for basic research
3. well-enforced patent protection
4. historically generous insurance (third party) payers
5. extensively subsidized employer-based private insurance for the majority of its citizens
6. physicians and hospitals that are motivated to use the highest technology available (Johnson-Lans, 2004)

TECHNOLOGICAL DIFFUSION

The United States ranks highly in the diffusion of most medical technologies. A study comparing this country with two other countries known for excellent health care, Canada and Germany, illustrates this (Rublee, 1994). The United States ranked highest in the diffusion of all technologies studied. The advantages were particularly large in the case of magnetic resonance imaging (MRI) and radiation therapy. Both of these technologies require very high levels of both physical and human capital investment. These examples illustrate the fact that use of advanced technologies requires complementary support in the form of well-equipped treatment centers and medical personnel with the specialized training to perform the procedures.

Factors that Promote Technological Diffusion

Economic incentives have been found to affect the rates of diffusion of new high technology treatments. In multicountry studies of the rate at which advanced technology treatments for heart attacks were adopted, higher rates of diffusion were found in countries with fee-for-service reimbursement systems—examples are Japan, Korea, Australia, and France. The United States, which has a blend of fee-for-service and prospective payment systems, was found to be experiencing an immediate rate of growth in the utilization of high technology treatments, although its stock of medical technology is still higher on a per capita basis than anywhere else in the world (McClellan, 2002).

MEASURING THE CONTRIBUTION OF TECHNOLOGICAL CHANGE

In empirical studies of healthcare costs, technological change has been treated as a residual that is left over as the unexplained variance after all known factors have been accounted for. This is known as the Solow residual. After sorting out the effects of other factors, technological change came to be widely regarded as the chief contributor to the increased expenditure on health care in the United States (Newhouse, 1993). More recently, Newhouse, Cutler, McClellan and others have developed an approach that measures technological change more directly (Cutler et al. 1999). Their approach can only be used to study the relationship between cost and technology change in treating specific diseases, such as coronary care.

Cost Increasing Versus Cost Saving Innovations

A cost-increasing innovation in medicine is an innovation that increases the cost of treatment for a particular disease. Where there is no incentive to contain costs, it may be more profitable for firms to develop more expensive or **cost-increasing technologies**. A number of economists argued that at least until the mid-1980s, both Medicare and the prevalent indemnity form of private insurance encouraged a bias toward cost-increasing (as well as quality increasing) innovation (Johnson-Lans, 2004).

It may be useful to distinguish between process and product innovations. Process innovations are often cost-saving. For example, the institution of more expensive and more efficacious new drugs has been shown to provide significant cost savings on nondrug expenditures that greatly outweigh the increase in the expenditure on drugs in the treatment of similar diseases (Lichtenberg, 2002). Using data from 1986 to 1998, the reduction in nondrug expenditures associated with the use of newer drugs was found to be on average 7.2 times the increase in the drug expenditures. For the Medicare population, the reduction in total expenditure on nondrug aspects of treatments, including both individual out-of-pocket expenditures and Medicare's contribution, was 8.3 times the increase in the expenditure on drugs (Lichtenberg, 2002). These are examples of unambiguous cost-saving improvements in technology.

An example of a cost-increasing innovation is laparoscopic cholecystectomy surgery to remove the gallbladder using a small inserted camera to direct the surgeon's instruments. It is particularly notable because of the rapid diffusion of this technique after it became available in the United States in the 1980s. By 1992, 80 percent of the cholecystectomies performed in this country were laparoscopic. The technique is more frequently used in the early stages of the disease among younger, non-Medicaid patients, but it has also come to be widely used among the elderly, including the very elderly for whom it is also appropriate and effective (Walling et al., 1999). The new technique has been shown to cut mortality rates in half for all age groups. Among the elderly, it has also greatly reduced the need for stays in skilled nursing homes. It has shortened average recovery time. Patients are also able to return to work in an average of 15 days as opposed to 31 days, and hospital stays have been reduced from 4.3 to 1.6 days (Johnson-Lans, 2004).

Even if the increase in the need for gallbladder surgery had not accompanied the development of the laparoscopic technique, the innovation defined narrowly, is more expensive. Even though hospital stays are shorter, total surgeon and hospital charges are higher for laparoscopic surgery than for open surgery and they outbalance savings in hospitalization costs (Johnson-Lans, 2004).

Certain stages in the development of medical treatments may tend to involve initially higher costs followed by lower costs. Therefore, it depends at what point in the life cycle of the innovation the costs are measured. Scientific discoveries often have life cycles that lead to first- and second-generation technological improvements. The two stages have been called halfway technologies and high technology by Weisbrod (1991). Halfway technologies are usually more expensive than cures and are certainly cost-increasing when compared to no treatment or watching and waiting during certain disease stages. Compare the early treatments for polio mellitus, a disease that was life-threatening well into the 1950s in high-income countries. The iron lung was an expensive machine that kept the paralyzed alive, but required intensive care. Contrast this with the second-generation innovation, the Salk and Sabine vaccines, which prevented the disease and were inexpensive and noninvasive. Here, the development of vaccines replaces expensive combinations of machinery and drugs (Johnson-Lans, 2004).

Productive Efficiency

Studies of alternative technologies used in the treatment of specific diseases often compare treatment methods in terms of their productive efficiency. **Productive efficiency** compacts the quantities of inputs used to produce a given output. Comparing production functions without reference to prices of inputs is a fairly standard way of making intercountry comparisons of the use of various medical technologies. For example, Bailey and Garber (1997) compared the United States,

Germany, and the United Kingdom in the treatments for diabetes, gallstones, breast cancer, and lung cancer. The United States was found to be more productively efficient than Germany in the treatment of each of the diseases except for diabetes, which requires long term therapies and little high technology.

The lack of capacity of capital equipment imposed by the British National Health Service budget limited the use of laparoscopic surgery. In Germany as well, these techniques were less prevalent than in the United States. This resulted in more time and resources to achieve better or worse outcomes. Productive efficiency is therefore not independent of previous decisions made in several countries about how much to allocate to developing capital capacity and technology (Johnson-Lans, 2004).

In the treatment of breast cancer, the United States and United Kingdom were both unambiguously more productive than Germany. The United States achieved a 9 percent better outcome using 38 percent fewer inputs and the United Kingdom achieved a 6 percent better outcome using 53 percent fewer resources. Compared to the United Kingdom, the United States used 15 percent more inputs to achieve a 3 percent better outcome (Bailey and Garber, 1997).

SUMMARY

The United States still leads the world in the introduction of healthcare technology in spite of cost-containment policies on the part of government and private managed care insurers. In the best-case scenario, cost-containment will tip the balance toward "cost-saving" technologies, but not significantly reduce the rate of innovation.

Key Words

- Intellectual property rights
- Cost-increasing technology
- Productive efficiency

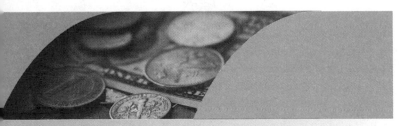

Questions

1. How would you characterize the effect of the United States health insurance system on health-care technology changes from 1960 to 1990?

2. How may the way in which providers are reimbursed affect the diffusion of technology?

REFERENCES

1. Bailey, MN and AM Garber. (1997) Health care productivity. *Brookings Papers on Economic Activity: Microeconomics*, 143–202.

2. Baker, LC and J Spetz. (1999) *Managed Care and Medical Technology Growth*. NBER Working Paper No. 6894. Cambridge, MA: National Bureau of Economic Research.

3. Cooke, P. (2001) Biotechnology clusters in the UK: lessons from the localisation in commercialisation of science. *Small Business Economics*, 17:58.

4. Cutler, D, McClellan, M, and J Newhouse. The costs and benefits of intensive treatment of cardiovascular disease. In: Triplett, J, ed. *Measuring the Price of Medical Treatments*. Washington, DC: Brookings Institution Press; 1999.

5. Johnson-Lans, S. (2004) *A Primer for Health Economics*. Boston: Pearson Addison Wesley.

6. Lichtenberg, F. (2002) *Benefits and Costs of Newer Drugs: An Update*. NBER Working Paper No. 8996. Cambridge, MA: National Bureau of Economic Research.

7. MacPherson, A. (2002) The contribution of academic industry interaction to product innovation: The case of New York State's medical devices sector. *Regional Science*, 81:121–129.

8. McClellan, MB et al. Technological change in heart attack care in the United States. In: McClellan, MB and DP Kessler, eds. *Technological Change in Health Care: A Global Analysis of Heart Attack*. Ann Arbor: University of Michigan Press; 2002.

9. McRae, JJ and F Tapon. (1985) Some empirical evidence on postpatent barriers in the Canadian pharmaceutical industry. *Journal of Health Economics*, 4:43–61.

10. Newhouse, JP. (1992) Medical care costs: How much welfare loss? *Journal of Economic Perspectives*, 6:3–22.

11. ———— (1993) *Free for All? Lessons from the RAND Health Insurance Experiment*. Cambridge, MA: Harvard University Press.

12. Rublee, DA. (1994) Medical technology in Canada, Germany and the United States: An update. *Health Affairs*, 13:113–117.

13. Schumpeter, JA. (1942) *Capitalism, Socialism, and Democracy*. New York: Harper.

14. Walling, AD et al. (1999) Laparoscopic Cholecystectomy vs. open surgery in the elderly. *American Family Physician*, 59:2321.

15. Weisbrod, BA. (1991) The health care quadrilemma: An essay on technological change, insurance, quality of care and cost containment. *Journal of Economic Literature*, 29:523–552.

BIO: PAUL J. FELDSTEIN

Paul J. Feldstein shares the sentiment of hundreds of graduates of one of the most prestigious economics departments in the country—the University of Chicago. He feels that health legislation arises from people acting in their own economic self interest rather than on the common notion of altruism and the concern for the indigent which are driving forces behind the healthcare reform movement.

Feldstein received his PhD from the University of Chicago in 1961 and spent the first three years of his professional career as the director of research for the American Hospital Association. He then moved to join the faculty of the University of Michigan. In 1987, he moved to the University of California at Irvine, where he is currently a professor and Robert Gumbiner Chair in Health Care Management.

Feldstein has served as principal investigator on 11 research grants. During several academic leaves of absence, he has served as a consultant with the Office of Management and Budget, the Social Security Administration, the World Health Organization, and the National Bureau of Economic Research. He regularly serves as an expert witness in legal cases involving healthcare antitrust issues.

Author of six books and more than 60 journal articles on healthcare issues, Feldstein's current research interests focus on the cost-containment strategies used by insurance companies. He has had a profound influence on students of economics worldwide, primarily through his book *Health Care Economics* (Delmar Publishers, Inc, 1999). First published in 1973, this book has been required reading for almost three decades for an entire generation of health economics students.

Source: Health Economics and Policy, 2nd Edition. James W. Henderson. (Cincinnati, OH: South-western, 2002).

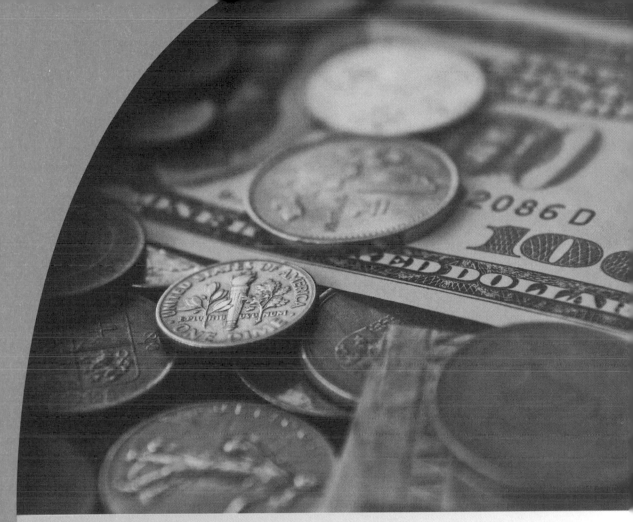

PART IV

HEALTHCARE MARKETS

The Competitive Market

THE PERFECTLY COMPETITIVE MARKET

The characteristics of perfect competition are many sellers possessing tiny market shares, a homogeneous product, no barriers to entry, and perfect consumer information. There is substantial actual competition because there are many substitute firms offering identical products. The potential for competition also exists because nothing prevents new firms from entering the industry. For example, a single supplier of alcohol swabs may be reluctant to increase price if the resulting higher profits entice new firms offering alcohol swabs to enter the market. The high degree of both actual and potential competition in a perfectly competitive market means that one firm's production decision has no meaningful impact on the overall performance of the industry. Therefore, the individual firm has no market power.

Is a Perfectly Competitive Market Relevant in Health Care?

People who have had little exposure to the study of economics tend to have different ideas about what perfect competition entails. Perfect competition is an abstract model and encompasses the four assumptions noted above. It also involves the assumptions of utility and profit maximization that underlie conventional microeconomic analysis. If any one of the assumptions is violated, firms and markets are unlikely to behave as the perfectly competitive market model predicts (Johnson-Lans, 2004).

When applied to healthcare industries, many of the assumptions of microeconomic analysis and characteristics of perfect competition often do not fit well. Several examples highlight this point. First, the nonprofit status of medical firms means that healthcare providers may not pursue maximum economic profits. Second, licensure creates a barrier to entry and decreases potential competition. Third, consumers typically lack perfect information about prices and technical aspects of medical services, which may lead to physicians practicing opportunistically.

While deviations from the characteristics of perfect competition and assumptions of microeconomic theory may make it inappropriate to use the model to evaluate the healthcare markets, the perfect competition model fulfills several important purposes. First, supply and demand, which are based on perfect competition, are useful in determining the impacts of market changes on price and output—even in medical markets. Second, healthcare markets may be reasonably competitive so supply and demand frameworks are appropriate. Third, the perfectly competitive market can serve as a gold standard to which other market models can be compared in terms of changes in prices and outputs (Johnson-Lans, 2004).

Supply and Demand

Perfect competition is based on a model where a large number of consumers and producers maximize their own personal utilities and profits, respectively. The massive number of participants in the market leads to everyone being a price taker because no individual has influence over the market. To maximize utility, each consumer consumes goods or services to the point that **marginal private benefit** (*MPB*) equals price. The profit-maximizing firm will produce up to the point where **marginal private cost** (*MPC*) equals price. The market clearing process occurs when the *MPC* equals the *MPB*, with price being the coordinating device ($MPB = P = MPC$). This can be shown graphically.

Suppose supply and demand in Figure 9-1 represents the market for generic antidepressants. The per-unit price of the generic is shown on the vertical axis and the quantity, *q*, is shown on the horizontal axis. The market demand curve, *D*, is downward sloping, reflecting the substitution and income effects seen with a lower price for a product. The demand curve also shows the diminishing *MPB* of consuming additional units of the generic drug. The supply curve, *S*, is upward sloping, showing that the *MPC* is increasing with the production of additional units of the drug. *MPC* reflects the variable costs of producing the good or service, which include the costs of labor and the materials needed. *MPC* increases in the short run because there is a capacity constraint caused by a fixed input, such as the equipment or size of the facility. Because of the higher *MPC*, a higher price is needed to encourage additional production of the drug. The market supply curve is derived by horizontally summing across all firms the portion of the marginal cost curve that lies above the minimum point of the average variable cost curve (Johnson-Lans, 2004).

In equilibrium, or the market clearing condition, price and output of the drug are at the point where demand intersects supply or where quantity demanded equals quantity supplied. By definition, equilibrium occurs when there is no tendency to change. At P_0 consumers are willing and able to purchase q_0 units of the drug because that represents the utility-maximizing amount. In addition, producers of the drug which provide q_0 units on the market at this price because that is the profit-maximizing amount. Therefore, both consumers and producers are perfectly satisfied with the exchange because both can purchase or sell their desired quantities at a price of P_0. The area under the demand curve above Price, P_0, (P_0AE_0) measures consumer surplus, which reflects the net benefit to consumers from engaging in free exchange. Consumer surplus shows the difference between what a consumer is willing to pay and what the consumer actually pays for some level of output. Analogously, the area below price but above the supply curve (BP_0E_0) represents the producer surplus, which is the net benefit to producers from free trade. Producer surplus measures the difference between the actual price received by the seller and the required price as reflected by the *MPC* for each additional unit produced. The sum of the consumer and producer surplus is the total net gains from trade for the consumers and producers (Johnson-Lans, 2004).

An inefficient allocation of resources may result in a perfectly competitive market when others, in addition to the market participants, are affected positively or negatively by the market exchange. Inefficiency results from the fact that utility-maximizing consumers and profit-maximizing producers only focus on the *MPB* and *MPC*, respectively—and not the full social impacts of their actions. It is likely that allocative efficiency results for the generic antidepressant market example because others besides the consumers and producers of the drug are unaffected by the exchange.

Comparative Statics

The demand and supply framework can be used to examine how surpluses and shortages of goods and services can occur and to study changes in prices and quantities of goods and services in various markets. **Comparative static** analysis examines how changes in market conditions influence the positions of the demand and supply curves and cause the equilibrium price and quantity to change. As the demand and supply curves shift, we can chart the price and output effects by comparing the different equilibria. Comparative statics can be used to explain effects of market changes in the past or predict future outcomes.

Several factors, such as the number of buyers, consumer tastes, income, and the price of substitutes and complements, affect the position of the market demand curve. Analogously, factors such as the input prices, technology, and number of producers affect the position of the supply curve by impacting the cost of production. A change in any one of these factors shifts the corresponding curve and alters the price and output of goods and services in the market (Johnson-Lans, 2004).

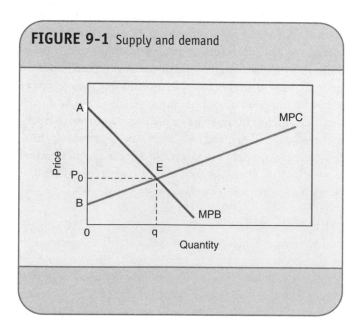

FIGURE 9-1 Supply and demand

For example, suppose that the number of producers has increased for the production of generic antidepressants, so that it is cheaper to produce the product at every price. This would cause a shift outward of the supply curve for a given demand curve. In Figure 9-2, note that this causes a temporary surplus of EF in the market as price remains constant. A surplus develops because at the initial price, the quantity supplied on the new supply curve, S1, is greater than the quantity demanded at that price. However, price does not remain constant in a competitive market and is eventually lowered from P_0 to P_1. The lower price creates an incentive for consumers to purchase more of the drug in the market, and quantity demanded increases from q_0 to q_1. Therefore, under normal conditions, supply and demand models predict that a lower price and higher quantity of the drug are associated with improved technology, all else being constant (Johnson-Lans, 2004).

Note that price serves several important functions. First, price provides useful information to both consumers and producers regarding the relative availability and value of a good or service in the market. Second, price serves as a coordination device, by bringing actions of consumers and producers into harmony and creating market clearing conditions. Third, price serves as a rationing device, distributing the goods and services to consumers who value them most. Fourth, price acts as incentive mechanism, encouraging more resources to markets with shortages and fewer resources to markets with surpluses.

Market Entry and Exit

As noted above, firms may enter the industry as changes in profits in various markets occur. For example, because there are no barriers to entry in a perfectly competitive market, excess profits create an incentive for new firms to enter an industry as they strive to make higher-than-normal rates of return. On the other hand, economic losses create an incentive for firms to leave an industry to avoid an unusually low rate of return on their investment.

When long run normal profits exist in a perfectly competitive industry, the market is in long run equilibrium, with firms having no incentive to enter or exit the industry. Normal profits result when the revenue generated just covers the opportunity costs of every input, including the normal return to capital.

Long run entry in response to excess profits can be treated as shifting the short run supply curve to the right. Analogously, long run exit causes the short run supply curve to shift to the left. For a given demand curve, these adjustments in the short run supply curve create a change in the price of the good and eventually restore normal profits. Because of entry and exit in the market, it is expected that the typical perfectly competitive firm earns a normal profit in the long run.

The importance of entry and exit in a market can be seen as follows. Entry of new firms leads to greater allocation of resources in response to favorable profit opportunities. Analogously, exit of firms helps to eliminate excess resources and producers from the market, creating greater efficiency. Profits serve as an important incentive mechanism and bring about an efficient allocation of resources in the long run. Free entry and exit of firms can occur only in perfectly competitive markets because barriers to entry and exit are nonexistent (Johnson-Lans, 2004).

SUMMARY

In this chapter, perfect competition in health care is examined. Perfect competition means that individual firms are price takers and maximize profits, consumers maximize utility, no barriers to entry or exit exist, and consumers have perfect information. Based on these characteristics, it can be shown that a perfectly competitive market allocates resources efficiently when all social costs and benefits are internalized by those engaged in the market. In other words, no externalities exist. Another sign of allocative efficiency is seen in the maximization of producer and consumer surplus.

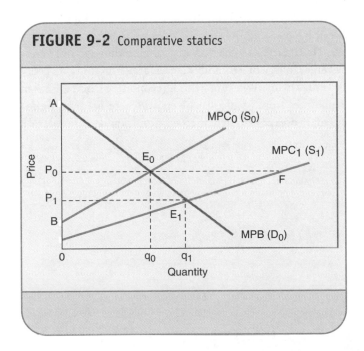

FIGURE 9-2 Comparative statics

Key Words

- Marginal private benefit
- Marginal private cost
- Comparative statics

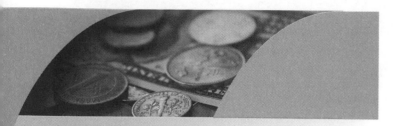

Questions

1. Suppose that the supply curve of healthcare services is perfectly inelastic (i.e., vertical). Analyze the impact of an increase in consumer income on the market price and quantity of the services. Now, suppose that the demand for healthcare services is perfectly inelastic (i.e., vertical), while the supply curve is upward sloping. Analyze the impact of an increase in input prices on the market price of healthcare services.

2. Suppose health insurance is nonexistent and all medical markets are perfectly competitive. Use supply and demand analysis to explain the impact of the following changes on the price and output of physician services:

    a. a decrease in the wage of clinic based nurses
    b. the adoption of cost-saving medical technology
    c. declining consumer income
    d. a lower market price for physician services

REFERENCE

1. Johnson-Lans, S. (2004) *A Primer for Health Economics*. Boston: Pearson Addison Wesley.

BIO: MICHAEL CHERNEW

Michael Chernew, PhD, is a professor in the Department of Health Care Policy at Harvard Medical School. One major area of his research focuses on assessing the impact of managed care on the healthcare marketplace, with an emphasis on examining the impact of managed care on healthcare cost growth and on the use of medical technology. Other research has examined determinants of patient choice of hospital and the impact of health plan performance measures on employee and employer selection of health plans.

Dr. Chernew is a member of the Commonwealth Foundation's Commission on a High Performance Health Care System. In 2000 and 2004, he served on technical advisory panels for the Center for Medicare and Medicaid Services that reviewed the assumptions used by the Medicare actuaries to assess the financial status of the Medicare trust funds. On the panels, Dr. Chernew focused on the methodology used to project trends in long-term healthcare cost growth. In 1998, he was awarded the John D. Thompson Prize for Young Investigators by the Association of University Programs in Public Health. In 1999, he received the Alice S. Hersh Young Investigator Award from the Association of Health Services Research. Both of these awards recognize overall contributions to the field of health services research. Dr. Chernew is a research associate of the National Bureau of Economic Research and is on the editorial boards of Health Affairs and Medical Care Research and Review. He is also coeditor of the *American Journal of Managed Care* and senior associate editor of *Health Services Research*.

Dr. Chernew received an AB from the University of Pennsylvania College of Arts and Sciences, a BS from the University of Pennsylvania Wharton School (economics), and a PhD in economics from Stanford University, where his training focused on areas of applied microeconomics and econometrics.

Source: Harvard University Web site.

Market Failures and the Role of Government

PARETO EFFICIENCY

In the real world, most healthcare markets rarely, if ever, achieve Pareto efficiency. According to Pareto, an economically efficient outcome in society is one under which it is impossible to improve the situation of any person without hurting someone else. Pareto efficiency also implies that no further exchanges can be found that improve the situation of everyone to some degree (Folland et al., 2007). For example, the First Fundamental Theorem of Welfare Economics relies crucially on markets being perfectly competitive—any breakdown in the underlying assumptions, such as freedom of market entry and exit, will lead to distortions in prices, quantities, and social efficiency. The First Fundamental Theorem states that competitive markets under certain conditions are economically efficient (Folland et al., 2007). The term "market failure" is used to cover all circumstances in which Pareto efficiency is not achieved by the market. The main causes of market failure in health care are described following.

EXTERNALITIES

Externalities, or spillover effects, are costs and benefits incurred in the consumption or production of goods and services that are not borne by the individual consumer or producer. The spillover effects can be positive or negative. Whenever other members of society are affected beneficially by a spillover effect, there is said to be external benefits. Whenever other members of society are affected adversely there are external costs.

Healthcare markets will not lead to Pareto efficiency if there are externalities. In other words, the full marginal costs to society from the production or consumption of health care (SMC) is equal to the private marginal cost (PMC) plus the marginal external cost (MEC); and the marginal benefit to society (SMB) is equal to the private marginal benefit (PMB) plus the marginal external benefit (MEB). Therefore, consumption and production decisions made in the market, which are based on private marginal benefits and costs, will not equal social marginal costs and benefits if the marginal external cost or the marginal external benefit is nonzero (Morris et al., 2007).

There are four types of externalities:

1. External Costs of Production ($MEC > 0$; $SMC > PMC$)

External costs of production might arise if a firm producing pharmaceuticals dumps its waste in a river or pollutes the air. In this case, the pollution caused by the firm will impose a positive external cost on society.

2. External Benefits of Production ($MEB > 0$; $SMB > PMB$)

Imagine a pharmaceutical firm undertaking research to identify a new compound to bring to market. If a promising compound is discovered, this will eventually lead to the publication of scientific papers on the properties of the compound. Patent laws prevent other firms from copying the product, but the research undertaken by the firm may identify useful avenues of research for other firms. In this case, there may be external benefits of production arising from research and development.

3. External Costs of Consumption ($MEC<0$; $SMC<PMC$)

The consumption of cigarettes and alcohol may lead to external costs of consumption. In addition to their effects on individual health, their consumption may also have negative effects on the rest of society in terms of passive smoking and antisocial behavior.

4. External Benefits of Consumption ($MEB>0$; $SMB>PMB$)

Public health interventions, such as vaccines, may have external benefits of consumption. This is because they can have a direct health benefit to others by reducing their chances of ill health. Whenever there are external benefits, there will be too little consumed or produced in the market. Whenever there are external costs, there will be too much consumed or produced in the market.

PUBLIC GOODS

Public goods are goods which may be jointly consumed by everyone. Specifically, public goods have two characteristics. The first is nonrivalry. This means that the consumption of a good or service by one individual will not prevent the consumption of the same good or service by others. The implication is that nonrival goods tend to have large marginal external benefits, which makes them socially very desirable, but privately unprofitable to provide. Commonly-used examples of nonrival goods include street lighting and pavement.

The second characteristic is nonexcludability. This means that it is not possible to provide a good or service to one individual without letting others also consume it. That is, it is not possible to exclude others from consumption. Nonexcludability means that individuals can obtain the benefits from consuming a nonexcludable good without paying for it. Because there is no incentive for individuals to pay for nonexcludable goods, this leads to a free-rider problem, in which individuals are unwilling to pay for goods and services if other people are willing to pay for them. The implication is that if everyone free-rides, then the good or service will not be provided at all, which might lead to a loss to society. Examples of nonexcludable goods include lighthouses and national defense (Johnson-Lans, 2004).

When goods have these features they will not be provided in the private market. This is because there is no incentive for private people to pay for them. Generally, public goods are provided by the government, which then compels individuals to finance their provision via some form of taxation. Note the distinction between public goods, which are nonrival and nonexcludable goods or services, and publicly-provided goods, which are goods and services that are provided by the government.

Pareto efficiency requires that the level of provision of a public good occurs where $SMB=SMC$. Because public goods are jointly consumed, the social marginal benefit (SMB) is obtained by summing the private marginal benefits across all individuals. Because people will free-ride, the good will be provided by the government and the individuals will be compelled to pay the price via taxation (Johnson-Lans, 2004).

Most healthcare products and services are not public goods because they are both rival and excludable. The receipt of health care by one person will usually exclude another person from consuming the same health care at that time. For example, one person's admission to a hospital bed prevents another from using the same bed. However, there are some healthcare programs that do have public good properties. An example is public health interventions aimed at preventing the spread of bird flu (Morris et al., 2007).

INFORMATION IMPERFECTIONS

Market failure also arises in health care due to imperfect information. These arise in health care due to uncertainty and to imperfect knowledge. Certainty in healthcare markets implies that buyers know exactly what health care they wish to consume, when they want to consume it, and how they can obtain it. Certainty is required for Pareto efficiency because consumers need to know the quantity of health care they would like to demand and providers need to know the quantity of health care to provide. If consumers have certainty, they are able to budget their finances in order to be able to afford their consumption. With uncertainty, a market is unable to function properly because consumers and producers do not know how much of a good to demand and supply. They are therefore unable to equate the private marginal benefits with the private marginal cost (Johnson-Lans, 2004).

The assumption of certainty may hold for certain aspects of health care. For example, pregnancies may be planned and it is possible to predict the timing of a birth and the cost of healthcare services required. Therefore, consumers of maternity services will know how much health care to demand and providers will know how much health care to supply. However, the consumption of the majority of healthcare services cannot be planned in this way. This is because illness and deteriorations in health are often sudden and unexpected. Therefore, there is uncertainty in the market and the demand for health care cannot be predicted in advance. Unless consumers and producers are well informed, they may take actions that are not in their best interests and they will be unable to equate private marginal benefits with private marginal costs, and therefore private efficiency (and thus, Pareto efficiency) is unlikely to be achieved.

The assumption of perfect knowledge on the part of consumers means that they are aware of their health status and of all the options open to them to maintain or improve their health. Although this may be the case for some illnesses, it is clearly not the case for the majority. Therefore, the market for health care is characterized by imperfect knowledge. Unfortunately, perfect knowledge is especially important in the market for health care because making the wrong decision can have much more serious consequences than the decision whether or not to, for example, consume a meal (Johnson-Lans, 2004).

THE MONOPOLY MODEL

If a firm has some market power, the competitive model is not appropriate and a noncompetitive model should be used. The difference between the two models concerns how the individual firm treats market price. In a perfectly competitive market, the individual firm is a price taker. That is, price is beyond the control of a single firm so each time a perfectly competitive firm sells an additional unit of output, market price measures the additional revenue received. Economists refer to **marginal revenue** (*MR*) as the additional revenue generated from selling one more unit of a good or service. Therefore, $P = MR$ for a price taker. A noncompetitive firm with some degree of market power, in contrast, faces a downward-sloping demand curve and therefore has some ability to influence the market price. To illustrate how a noncompetitive model can be used to examine firm behavior, a pure monopoly is first considered, which is the opposite of a perfectly competitive market. A pure monopoly is a market where only one producer of a good or service is in the market (Johnson-Lans, 2004).

Monopoly Compared to Perfect Competition

A monopoly is the sole provider of a good or service in a well-defined market with no close substitutes. Because it is the only seller in the market, it faces the market demand curve, which is always downward sloping due to substitution and income effects associated with a price change. Given the downward sloping demand, the only way a monopolist can sell more of the good or service is to lower the price of the product.

Assuming that price is the same for all units sold at a point in time, price must be lowered not only for the next unit, but for all previous units as well. Due to this, marginal revenue will be less than price at each level of output. For a linear demand curve, it can be shown that marginal revenue has the same intercept, but twice the slope of the demand curve. Suppose the inverse demand is $P = a - bQ$. Total revenue equals PxQ or $(a - bQ)Q = aQ - bQ^2$. Taking the first derivative of this revenue function with respect to Q will result in $dTR/dQ = MR = a = 2bQ$. This MR function has the same intercept as the demand function (i.e., a), and twice the slope (i.e., $2bQ$) (Johnson-Lans, 2004).

Figure 10-1 can be used to show how the equilibrium price and quantity for a monopolist compare to the market price and quantity for a perfectly competitive market. As before, we can look at the market for generic antidepressants. The market demand for the drug is *AD*. The supply curve is labeled *GS* and reflects the *MPC* of producing the drug. Point *C* represents equilibrium in a perfectly competitive market, where supply and demand curves intersect. The market price and output of the drug equal *PC* and *QC*, respectively (Johnson-Lans, 2004).

Now suppose only one firm produces and sells the drug in that same market. Perhaps natural economies of scale lead to a monopoly position. Further suppose that a barrier to entry

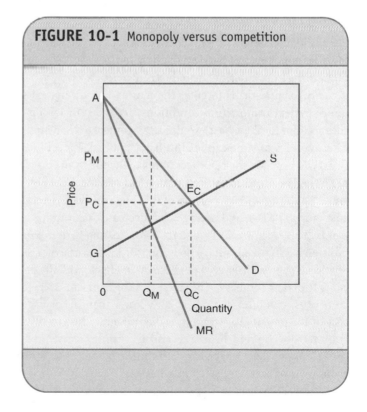

FIGURE 10-1 Monopoly versus competition

caused by the economies of scale prevents other firms from entering the market. The marginal revenue curve shares the same intercept as the demand curve, but has twice the slope. The monopolist chooses the price and quantity so that profits are maximized. Profit maximizing output occurs at Qm, where $MR = MC$ because producing and selling additional units of the drug always add to revenue more than costs up to that point. Beyond Q_m, production is unprofitable because marginal cost, MC, exceeds MR. Therefore, the monopoly outcome is represented by the point M and price charged equals P_m, which is derived from the demand curve for that particular output level.

Notice that the monopolist charges a higher price and a lower quantity of the drug than under the perfectly competitive conditions. Also note that the consumer surplus is reduced under the monopoly structure, but the producer surplus is increased. The rectangular area, reflects the surplus that is transferred from consumers to producers in a market that is controlled by a monopoly. There is also deadweight loss produced by the monopoly (denoted by the triangle). Deadweight loss shows that the value of the units no longer produced is greater than the opportunity costs of the resources used to produce them. This implies that the monopoly underproduces the drug and therefore misallocates society's scarce resources. The cost of the monopoly shows up in the deadweight loss (Johnson-Lans, 2004).

Barriers to Entry

For a firm to maintain its market power for an extended period of time, some types of barriers to entry must exist to prevent other firms from entering the industry. Barriers to entry make it costly for new firms to enter the market and do not exist under perfect competition conditions. Technical or legal issues account for these barriers. Exclusive control over an input or economies of scale can lead to barriers because the other firms will not have the resources to make the substitute product. When production exhibits economies of scale, a firm operates on the downward portion of the **long run average total cost** curve (*LATC*), and average cost decreases as output expands. This is shown in Figure 10-2. An existing firm in this position has a cost advantage that results from the scale of production. Potential firms cannot effectively compete with the existing firm on a cost basis. The larger existing firm with average costs of C_1 could set its price slightly lower than the average cost of the potential entrant, thus discouraging the potential entrant from entering the market and also gaining excess profits. Pricing to deter entry is called limit pricing. Therefore, economies of scale can serve as a barrier to entry that insulates the existing firm from potential competitors. Price regu-

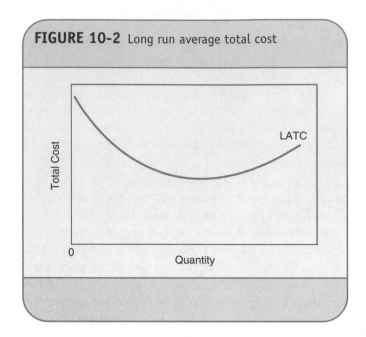

FIGURE 10-2 Long run average total cost

lations are often put into place when a firm has a monopoly structure from this position (Johnson-Lans, 2004).

Legal restrictions that prevent other firms from entering the market and providing goods or services similar to the existing firms are also barriers to entry. Patents on pharmaceutical products, occupational licensing, and other laws are examples of legal entry barriers in healthcare markets.

MONOPOLISTIC COMPETITION

In the monopolistically competitive structure, there are many firms with minimal barriers to entry. The main distinguishing characteristic of this market model is that firms sell differentiated products. Product differentiation is a result of advertising, real or perceived quality differences, or preferred location. Due to this differentiation, each firm faces a slightly elastic downward sloping demand curve. Because the demand curve is downward sloping, the firm can have a limited ability to raise prices without losing market share. Product differentiation leads to brand loyalty, which allows the firm to raise the price and continue to sell the product. All else constant, a more differentiated product leads to a less elastic demand curve facing the firm (Johnson-Lans, 2004).

Figure 10-3 shows the model of a profit-maximizing monopolistically competitive firm. The elasticity of the demand curve reflects the number of relatively imperfect substitutes for its product. Paxil may be a good example of a branded product that faces a downward sloping demand. Paxil, an antidepressant, has some generic competitors such as the generic for Zoloft, but the manufacturer can charge a higher price because it has a brand name. Given the linear demand, the *MR* is drawn with the same intercept as the demand curve, but with twice the slope. The long run *ATC* and *MC* curves denote all economies and diseconomies of scale (Johnson-Lans, 2004).

Given the downward sloping demand, the individual firm can earn an economic profit in the short run if the price charged is greater than the average total cost at the level of output where $MR=MC$. However, the limits on barriers to entry lead to the long run normal profits for this market model. Over time, other firms are attracted to the industry by the possibility of earning economic profits. As more firms enter the market, each firm sees its market share slowly diminish, which translates to a decreased demand for the product. The demand curve continues to shift to the left for each firm, resulting in prices declining to the point where economic profits equal zero, or price equals **average total costs** (*ATC*). Demand becomes more elastic and firms are no longer attracted to the industry. This results in economics profits in the long run to be zero.

Figure 10-3 shows the long run equilibrium in a monopolistically competitive market. The demand curve is tangent to the *ATC* where $MR=MC$. This implies that the firm earns zero economic profits in the long run because price equals *MC*, which is the same result as in the perfectly competitive case. However, the monopolistically competitive firm does not produce at a level where $P=MC$, as in the perfectly competitive model. This may imply that the monopolistically compet-

itive firm is producing output inefficiently, but this would best be determined by examining the costs and benefits of product differentiation (Johnson-Lans, 2004).

Competitive Aspects of Product Differentiation

In the perfectly competitive framework, consumers are treated as being perfectly informed about the prices and quantity of all goods and services in the market. The assumption concerning perfect information implies that all firms selling identical products sell at the same lowest possible price. Otherwise, firms with higher prices lose business to firms charging less when consumers are perfectly informed.

However, there are costs and benefits to acquiring information. In some situations, people choose to be less than perfectly informed, or rationally ignorant. Positive information costs may result in consumers being reluctant to seek out all available producers of a good or service. As a result, one individual producer faces a less than perfectly elastic demand curve and is able to restrict output and raise price to some extent to attain positive economic profits in the short run. As a result, the price of a good or service in the real world is likely to be dispersed and higher on average than in the perfectly competitive case. Higher benefits and lower costs of acquiring information result in lower price dispersion (Johnson-Lans, 2004).

Imperfect information may also affect the level of observed quality of goods and services in the market. Higher quality goods are produced at a higher price than lower quality goods. In a competitive market where consumers are perfectly informed, higher quality goods sell at a higher price than lower quality goods. In the real world with imperfect information, consumers are unsure about the exact quality of the goods and services under consideration. Therefore, if consumers base their information on the average quality in the market and pay the average price, lower quality goods and services drive out higher quality goods and services to the point where no products remain. This implies that the higher the level of quality of a good, the better informed the consumer group is.

Given imperfect information about many goods and services in the real world, some economists state that product differentiation, such as advertising and branding, can lead to improved information for the consumers. Some think that advertising about the quality and features of the good or service in question provides relatively cheap information about the good or service to the consumer, leading to lower prices and improved quality. Studies by Cady (1976) and Kwoka (1984) found that the prices of eyeglasses and prescription drugs were higher on average when advertising was prohibited. Even when price or quality information was not directly conveyed, a large

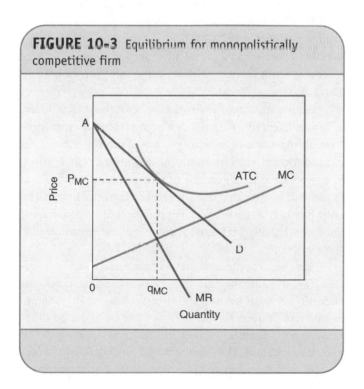

FIGURE 10-3 Equilibrium for monopolistically competitive firm

advertisement may provide a signal to consumers that the producer has a high quality product because the producer is confident to incur such a sizable expense. Through repeat purchases, the firm hopes to get a sufficient return on its advertising expenses. In this case, the presence of expensive advertising generates information about the quality of the product.

Other economists such as Klein and Leffler (1981) argue that branding can serve a similar purpose to advertising for promoting competition. Because many goods and services cannot be evaluated until after purchase, branding helps to identify firms that are confident enough to invest in establishing a reputation. The argument is that firms will not invest significant sums in branding their products only to have shoddy workmanship and a resulting tarnished reputation. This would result in a significant reduction in return on investment.

Some economists think that advertising and branding can lead to anticompetitive behavior through habit purchases rather than informed purchases, created through brand loyalty. Advertising in this argument is considered to be persuasive rather than informative. Sometimes the advertising points out real differences between products, but often the advertising is used to create perceived differences across goods or services. For example, Centrum and the generic brand of the vitamin contain the same active ingredients, yet many consumers are willing to pay the extra amount for the brand name. Some argue that consumers pay a premium for branded products because past advertising successfully convinced consumers that Centrum, for example, is a superior product. Instead of creating a new market demand, the advertising attempts to draw consumers away from the competitor (Johnson-Lans, 2004).

According to the anticompetitive viewpoint, product differentiation manipulates the demand for a product. Successful advertising can manipulate consumers' preferences, thus influencing the position of the demand curve for the product. The demand curve may shift up because consumers may be willing to pay more for the product, and the demand curve may become more inelastic with respect to price, giving the firm some ability to reduce output and raise price.

As an example, many public health professionals claim that the purpose behind cigarette advertising is to manipulate the demand for cigarettes. Of major concern is the advertising aimed at teenagers' demand for cigarettes. A report by the Centers for Disease Control and Prevention found that among smokers aged 12 to 18, preferences were greater for Marlboro, Newport, and Camel, three brands that are heavily advertised (Ruffenach, 1992).

Existing firms may also use advertising or other types of product differentiation to create barriers to entry. If existing firms control the market through advertising, new firms may find it difficult to enter the market because they are unable to sell a sufficient amount of output to break even financially. It implies that product differentiation aimed at creating artificial wants, habit buying, or barriers to entry, results in the misallocation of resources. Resources are misused if they are employed to create perceived rather than real value.

When evaluating the social desirability of product differentiation, most consumers like diversity and enjoy choosing among a wide variety of goods and services selling at different money and time prices. In this scenario, the higher than competitive price that is paid for product differentiation may simply reflect the premium consumers pay for variety. If supply creates demand through product differentiation, some of society's scarce resources may be wasted (Johnson-Lans, 2004).

OLIGOPOLY

An oligopoly is a market model with a few large firms and relatively high barriers to entry. There may be a large number of firms in the industry, but the other firms may be small price takers, with limited market share. The dominant firms must be sufficiently sized and limited in number so that the pricing or output decisions of one firm affect the same types of decisions for the other dominant firms in the market. This mutual interdependence among the firms distinguishes the oligopoly structure from other market models. This mutual interdependence varies and results in no one model of oligopoly behavior.

According to the collusive oligopoly model, all firms cooperate rather than compete on price and output and jointly maximize profits by collectively acting like a monopoly. It follows that a deadweight loss and misallocation of society's scarce resources result from a collusive oligopoly (Johnson-Lans, 2004).

Collusion among the firms may be overt or tacit. Overt collusion refers to a situation where representatives of firms formally meet, and coordinate prices and market shares. Tacit collusion occurs when firms informally coordinate their prices. Price leadership is an example of tacit collusion, where firms in the market agree that one firm will be the price maker. The other firms in the market match or parallel the price behavior of the leader. This market behavior can mimic the monopoly outcome as overt collusion.

There are a number of factors that make collusion difficult. First, there are the legal and practical considerations. The Sherman Antitrust Act prohibits overt collusion. Firms found in violation of overt pricing behavior can be subjected to severe financial penalties and the Chief Financial Officers (CFOs) may be imprisoned. However, antitrust officials do not pursue cases of tacit collusion, because there is the burden of proof.

Firms in a market may parallel their actions simply because they experience the same market shocks as other firms. However, a tacit collusive agreement has its own difficulties. Other firms may have difficulty interpreting price changes set by the leader. Also, cost differences make it more difficult for firms to cooperate and agree on a common price. High cost firms will desire a higher price than lower cost firms. However, the success of the collusion depends on the agreement on a common price. Collusion is also less successful when entry barriers are low. Lastly, collusion is more likely when only a few firms exist in the market. Low negotiation costs exist with fewer firms. Furthermore, the potential for cheating behavior is greater when more firms exist in the industry because of high monitoring costs. For these reasons, it is very difficult to form and maintain a collusive oligopoly structure (Johnson-Lans, 2004).

Competitive Oligopoly

Competitive oligopolies are where firms act competitively, do not cooperate, and seek to maximize their own profits. If the market consists of goods or services that are relatively homogeneous, firms will set the price equal to MC because there are many close substitutes for the product. With this pricing scheme, each firm will have some of the market share and will not be undersold. If firms behave in this way, market price equals MC, and resources are efficiently allocated—even though there are a few dominant firms in the market (Johnson-Lans, 2004).

THE ROLE OF GOVERNMENT

The public interest and special interest group theories describe the motivation behind government intervention in the healthcare market. The public interest theory states that the government intervenes in the best interest of society to promote efficiency and equity in the market. Recall that an efficient allocation of resources occurs when, for a given distribution of income, **marginal social benefit** is equal to **marginal social cost** ($MSB=MSC$). In the presence of market failures, such as imperfect information or monopolistic behaviors, markets fail to allocate resources efficiently.

The public interest is served when the government attempts to restore efficiency or to distribute income equitably by encouraging competition, providing information, reducing harmful externalities or redistributing income in society. Therefore, the public interest theory of government behavior predicts that the laws, regulations, and other government interventions enhance efficiency and equity (Johnson-Lans, 2004).

The special interest group theory (Becker, 1983) states that the political venue can be treated like any private market for goods and services so that amounts and types of legislation are determined by supply and demand for such legislation. Vote-maximizing legislators are the suppliers of legislation, while wealth-maximizing special interest groups are demanders of such legislation. In this structure, incumbent politicians increase the likelihood of getting reelected by moving wealth or resources away from the general public and moving them toward the powerful and influential special interest groups. In return, politicians expect votes, support, and political contributions. Professional lobbyists representing special interest groups negotiate with the legislators and arrive at market clearing types of legislation. This form of legislation changes over time with relative power shifts among different interest groups. Power or political pressure is determined by the amount of resources the group controls, the size of the group, and the efficiency with which the group transforms resources into pressure.

The successful politician stays in office by combining legislative programs of various special interest groups into an overall fiscal package to be advanced in the political arena. The beneficiaries are the special interest groups—the costs fall on the general public. Special interests forums and politicians are made better off by the legislation—otherwise it would not occur. The politicians retain or acquire elected positions and the special interest groups receive wealth enhancing legislation.

The general public is made worse off by the legislation. Individuals are rationally ignorant about the wealth implications of government activities because the cost of acquiring such information is high, and the private benefit is low. Moreover, the wealth transfer from the public to the special interest group is low in per capita terms. To challenge the special interest group legislation, a group or an individual must organize a legitimate counter political movement, inform others, circulate a petition, and engage in lobbying. All of these activities entail sizable personal and monetary costs.

The special interest group model of government behavior implies that the typical consumer is taken by wealth transfer ring legislation. The political negotiations leading to the wealth transfer involve scarce resources, such as a politician's time and professional lobbyists. As more resources are diverted to political negotiations, fewer resources are left for productive purposes. Therefore, inefficiencies are associated with this model.

Therefore, to protect the public, government intervention includes regulations and laws because some special interest group benefits at the expense of the general public. Individuals in a special interest group are collectively powerful because they share a common concentrated interest. Consumers as a group, however, are generally diverse and powerless. Organization and time costs prohibit the general public from taking action even when wealth transfers to the special interest groups are known.

The public interest and special interest group theories are contrasting models regarding the reasons why the government intervenes in a market-based system. In the real world, the government intervenes for two reasons. In some cases, market failures occur and the government intervenes to promote efficiency and equity. In other cases, government policies enhance the well-being of specific groups at an overall cost to society and therefore a misallocation of resources and inequitable distribution of income. It is important to remember that both the government and market can have imperfections or failures. In the real world, the role of informed consumers or analysts is to determine which institution can accomplish which objectives in the more equitable and efficient manner.

Forms of Government Intervention

The government can promote efficiency and equity by providing public goods, levying taxes, correcting for externalities, imposing regulations, enforcing antitrust laws, operating public enterprises, and sponsoring redistribution programs. As an example of a public good, a public health sanitation officer inspects the conditions at restaurants to protect the public's health. To correct for externalities, the government taxes the emissions of firms to reduce the level of air or water pollution in an area. The Sherman Act of 1890 prohibits independent physicians from discussing their pricing policies to prevent monopolistic practices, such as price fixing. A hospital operated by the Veterans' Administration is an example of government enterprise. Also, the social insurance programs of Medicaid and Medicare are examples of public medical care distribution programs. Each example influences the allocation of resources and the distribution of output in the healthcare economy (Johnson-Lans, 2004).

Antitrust Issues

Economists, and also courts dealing with antitrust cases, often use the concept of cross-price elasticity of demand to measure whether a firm has monopoly power in supplying a good or service in the given market. The cross-price elasticity of demand measures the degree to which the quantity demanded of a good X is related to the price of another good Y. It is defined as:

$$\frac{(\text{\% change in quantity of X demanded})}{(\text{\% change in price of Y})}$$

If the coefficient is negative, this provides evidence that the goods in question are complements, otherwise the goods are substitutes. If the coefficient of cross-price elasticity of demand for a good is positive and large enough in magnitude to be of some consequence, the firm probably does have effective monopoly power (Johnson-Lans, 2004).

The contemporary market for physician services provides some examples of behavior that we associate with collusive oligopoly or cartels, which are organizations that set output quotas and sometimes directly set prices. Examples of vertically- and horizontally-integrated networks of physicians have attained a virtual monopoly over local or even regional provision of physician services (Greenberg, 1998). Antitrust law allows clinically integrated groups to jointly contract. In ruling such cases, the Federal Trade Commission has argued that even if physician networks are not financially integrated, they can receive special treatment under the Rule of Reason (Johnson-Lans, 2004).

However, a series of Supreme Court decisions beginning in the 1970s, have interpreted antitrust law as applying to hospitals (Alpert and McCarty, 1984). The belief that consolidation was associated with lower costs was maintained by the courts throughout the 1970s and early 1980s (United States v. Carilion Health System and Community Hospital of Roanoke Valley). Since the late 1980s, the Justice Department has become critical of hospital mergers (Whitesell and Whitesell, 1995; Noether, 1998). Furthermore, government regulators have responded to the apparent change in the effects of concentration on hospital markets and now tend to see competition as beneficial. Difficulty in defining relevant geographic markets in which hospitals operate has led to very limited success on the part of the government in blocking large hospital mergers to date, but government policy remains suspicious of increasing concentration in the hospital sector.

Social Insurance Programs

The principles of social insurance are quite different from those that pertain to the private market. Social insurance programs are generally funded by mandatory contributions through some form of taxation. They usually have goals in addition to pooling of risk, which include transfers of benefits between groups, from the more affluent to the poor, from younger adults to senior citizens, from adults to children, or from the able-bodied to the disabled. Therefore, the goal is to equate marginal social benefits with marginal social costs in the provision of optimal insurance packages (Johnson-Lans, 2004).

Social insurance in the United States is limited to certain categories of citizens and residents, such as senior citizens, a segment of the poor, and people with qualified disabilities, all of whom are covered by Medicare and Medicaid. A few other special groups are covered by public insurance programs, including Native Americans on reservations, veterans of armed forces, members of Congress, and low-income families with children. Some states have also expanded social insurance programs to families who would not otherwise be covered by the federal programs.

Provision of Information

When market failure in health care arises due to imperfect information, the government may help to correct the problem via the provision of information. An example is the provision of information to the general public on the benefits of certain types of health care, such as the safety of the mumps, measles, and rubella (MMR) vaccine.

SUMMARY

The model of a pure monopoly is the exact opposite of the perfectly competitive market. This market model is characterized by one seller with one product and perfect barriers to entry. Due to the downward-sloping demand and the fact that the monopolist has market power, this results in the monopolist restricting output and a misallocation of society's resources.

Monopolistic competition is noted as an intermediate market model, with its main distinguishing feature being its differentiated product. Differentiated products allow the firm to raise price slightly without losing all market share. Because barriers to entry are nonexistent in the long run, the monopolistically competitive firm makes normal economic profits in the long run. Given that variety is valued by consumers, the only real criticism of this model is in the use of differentiation. If differentiation through branding, advertising, or trademark can provide cheap information and therefore a more competitive solution, it can also be argued that these same features can impede competition through brand loyalty and habitual buying behavior.

Oligopoly is also considered an intermediate market model. A few dominant firms and mutual interdependence between the firms distinguishes an oligopoly from the other market models. The efficiency of an oligopolistic market depends on the level of competition or cooperation among the firms in the market. Cooperation or collusion leads to monopolistic outcomes and a misallocation of resources. Competition leads to efficient allocation of resources.

Government intervention is based on the special interest or public interest theories. The public interest theory focuses on efficiency in the market and the special interest theory levels the playing field in the legislative marketplace.

Key Words

- Externalities
- Marginal revenue
- Long run average total cost
- Average total cost
- Marginal social benefit
- Marginal social cost

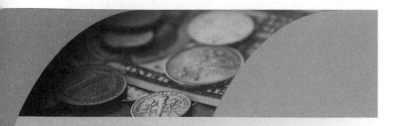

Questions

1. Show graphically and explain verbally how a monopoly results in deadweight loss. Also discuss the redistribution in society as a result of a monopoly.

2. Explain why economic profits are zero in the long run in a monopolistically competitive market.

3. What beneficial role do branding and trademarks serve when information imperfections exist?

4. Discuss the two ways that product differentiation affects the demand for the product.

5. Explain the difference between collusive and competitive oligopolistic market models.

6. What are the main differences between social and private insurance?

REFERENCES:

1. Alpert, G and TR McCarty. (1984) Beyond Goldfarb: Applying traditional antitrust analysis to changing health markets. *Antitrust Bulletin*, 29:165–204.

2. Becker, GS. (1983) Altruism in the family and selfishness in the market place. *Economics, New Series*, 4:1–15.

3. Cady, JF. (1976) An estimate of the price effects of restrictions on drug price advertising. *Economic Inquiry*, 14:473–510.

4. Folland, S, Goodman, AC, and M. Stano. (2007) *The Economics of Health and Health Care*, 5th ed. Upper Saddle River, NJ: Pearson/Prentice Hall.

5. Greenberg, W. (1998) Marshfield Clinic, physician networks and the exercise of monopoly power. *Health Services Research*, 33 Part 2:1461–1476.

6. Johnson-Lans, S. (2004) *A Primer for Health Economics*. Boston: Pearson Addison Wesley.

7. Klein, B and KB Leffler. (1981) The role of market forces in assuring contractual performance. *Journal of Political Economy*, 89:615–641.

8. Kwoka, JE. (1984) Advertising and the price and quality of optometric services. *American Economic Review*, 74(1):211–236.

9. Morris, S, Devlin, N, and D Parkin. (2007) *Economic Analysis in Health Care*. West Sussex, England: John Wiley & Sons, Ltd.

10. Noether, M. (1998) Economic issues of the antitrust assessment of hospital competition: overview. *International Journal of Economics and Business*, 5:133–141.

11. Ruffenach, G. (1992) Study says teenagers' smoking habits seem to be linked to heavy advertising. *The Wall Street Journal*, B8.

12. Whitesell, SE and WE Whitesell. (1995) Hospital mergers and antitrust: Some economic and legal issues. *American Journal of Economics and Sociology*, 54:305–321.

BIO: THOMAS G. MCGUIRE

Thomas G. McGuire, PhD, is a professor of health economics in the Department of Health Care Policy at Harvard Medical School. His research focuses on the design and impact of healthcare payment systems, the economics of healthcare disparities, and the economics of mental health policy. Dr. McGuire has contributed to the theory of physician, hospital, and health plan payment. His current research includes application of theoretical and empirical methods from labor economics to the area of healthcare disparities. He has analyzed the reasons behind "discrimination" by doctors, and conducted empirical research to identify the contribution of the various mechanisms behind healthcare disparities. For more than 25 years, Dr. McGuire has conducted academic and policy research on the economics of mental health.

Dr. McGuire was the 1981 recipient of the Elizur Wright Award from the American Association of Risk and Insurance for his book *Financing Psychotherapy*, and he has co-chaired four NIMH-sponsored conferences on the economics of mental health. He received the 1998 Arrow Award (joint with Albert Ma) from the International Health Economics Association. In 1991, he received the Carl Taube Award from the American Public Health Association. Dr. McGuire is a member of the Institute of Medicine, and a coeditor of the *Journal of Health Economics*.

Dr. McGuire received his BA degree from Princeton University and his PhD degree in economics from Yale University.

Source: Thomas G. McGuire curriculum vita. Harvard University Web site.

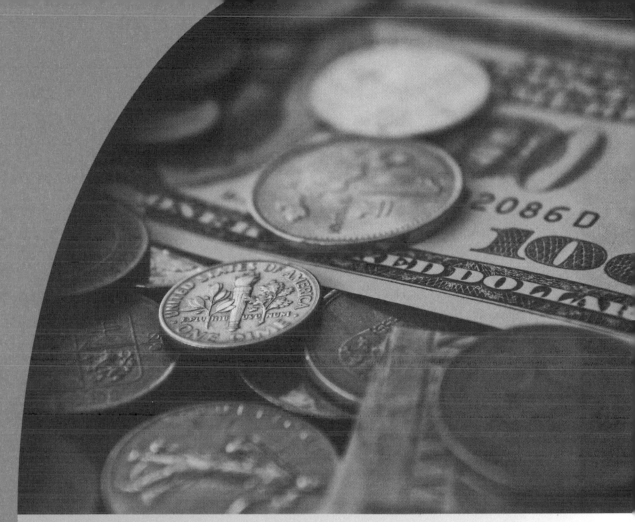

PART V

ISSUES IN HEALTH ECONOMICS

Socioeconomic Factors

SPENDING

The United States spends more on medical care than anyone else in the world, whether measured in total dollars spent, per capita expenditures, or as a share of GDP. For all of our spending it is unclear whether or not we are healthier than our foreign counterparts. Critics of the system say that life expectancy is lower than in other countries and the higher infant mortality may bolster their argument that the system is in need of a major overhaul.

TYPES OF SOCIETAL PROBLEMS

Two competing lines of thought address the nature of our society's problems: a liberal view and a conservative view. From the liberal viewpoint, social problems have their origin in the economy's inability to provide sufficient income-earning opportunities, especially for many males in lower socioeconomic classes. This premise usually leads to the recommendation that the government should become more involved in social programs ranging from direct welfare payments to various training and retraining efforts, which all require significant increases in federal budget outlays. The conservative viewpoint focuses on the breakdown of the traditional family values as the pri-

mary cause of our social pathologies, with the government as a significant contributor. Illegitimate births, single-parent families, and divorce lead to the phenomenon called the "feminization of poverty." Children raised under these circumstances are more likely to drop out of school, use drugs, and participate in illegal activity. This pattern of behavior is influenced by governmental involvement that creates incentives to reinforce these lifestyle choices. The purpose of this chapter is to examine the various social problems and pathologies and how they impact on the delivery of health care in the United States.

AIDS in the United States

More than 33 million people worldwide are infected with the human immunodeficiency virus (HIV) that causes **acquired immunodeficiency syndrome (AIDS)** and more that 16 million have already died as a result of complications from the

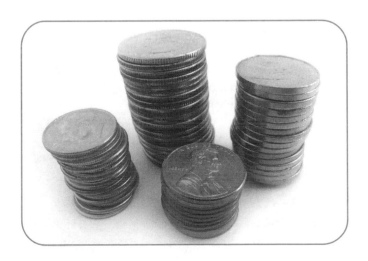

disease. By the end of 1999, almost 725,000 United States cases were reported to Centers for Disease Control (CDC) and 400,000 Americans died of the disease (CDC, 1999).

Acquired immunodeficiency syndrome results when the human immune system is so weakened by HIV that the body can no longer fight off serious infections. A weakened immune system makes a person susceptible to other diseases, such as yeast infections of the mouth and throat, herpes infections, pneumonia, tuberculosis, and a form of cancer called Kaposi's sarcoma, which produces purple blotches on the skin. Symptoms of AIDS usually include fever, diarrhea, weight loss, and enlarged lymph glands.

From 1981, when AIDS was first discovered in clinical studies, until mid-1999, approximately 688,000 cases were reported. The fatality rate for those infected is quite high, 58.8 percent for adults and 58.5 percent for children. About 35,000 new cases are now diagnosed annually in the United States (Henderson, 2002). Although half of the new cases afflict either homosexual or bisexual males, or intravenous (IV) drug users, transmission of the virus that causes AIDS has slowed dramatically in this segment of the population. Included in the 35,404 newly-reported cases involving adults and adolescents in 1998 were 268 cases involving children less than 13 years of age. Of this number, 232 were infected by their mothers who were also diagnosed with AIDS (CDC, 1999a).

At the end of 2000, over 300,000 Americans were living with AIDS, in addition to more that 113,000 diagnosed with severe HIV-related immunosuppression (CDC, 1999b). The evidence indicates that the rate of new cases has not spread much beyond the traditional risk groups, which includes hemophiliacs, transfusion recipients of blood or blood products, and perinatally-infected children of these categories. These groups now account for more than 85 percent of the total infections. Heterosexual contact cases of AIDS have not grown as rapidly as initially predicted. Only 66,489 cases have been reported to date, and more than 30,000 had equal partners who were members of traditional risk groups (Henderson, 2002).

Centers for Disease Control research estimated that nearly one-half of all new HIV infections are occurring in the drug injecting population (Holmberg, 1996). Changing the behavior of IV drug users represents the biggest challenge in the battle to control the spread of the disease. Unsafe practices, such as sharing needles and promiscuous sex, are the leading causes of infection. The extent of the problem may be greatly expanded if drug use increases substantially.

Risk to the Population

In 1991, the sports world was shocked by the revelation that one of its superstars, Ervin "Magic" Johnson, had tested positive for HIV. This was a lesson for the heterosexual population that anyone can be at risk. It is true that AIDS shows no respect for age, race, gender, or socioeconomic status. In that sense, we are all at risk. However, it is also true that we are not all *equally* at risk of contracting the deadly virus.

The transmission of the AIDS virus is primarily an inner-city problem that affects the minority community disproportionately and especially the intravenous drug-using segment of that community. By the end of 1999, more than half of the new cases were among African Americans, Latinos, and other minorities. The rate of cases per 100,000 people is seven times greater among blacks and two times greater among Hispanics than among whites (Henderson, 2002).

The vast majority of AIDS cases are reported in the large urban centers, such as San Francisco, Los Angeles, Dallas, Houston, New Orleans, Chicago, Atlanta, Philadelphia, Newark, New York, Boston, Miami, and the District of Columbia. In fact, more that 60 percent of all cases originated in the five states of New York, California, Florida, Texas, and New Jersey. Second, the incidence of AIDS is highest among minority groups, especially African Americans and Puerto Rican Hispanics. Black children constitute approximately 12 percent of the United States population of all children under the age of 13 with AIDS and most were infected prenatally (CDC, 1999b).

For the heterosexual community, the most important risk factor is the identity of the potential sex partners. If your sex partner has never been an IV drug user or the sex partner of an IV drug user and is not from the African or Caribbean countries where the disease is spread primarily through heterosexual contact, the chances of getting AIDS through heterosexual contact is 1 in 50,000. When the analysis is restricted to only the white population, the risk is reduced to 1 in 500,000 (Henderson, 2002).

Prostitute hemophiliacs are considered to be primary sources of the transmission of AIDS into the heterosexual community. However, fewer than 3 percent of all reported cases in the United States are a result of someone outside a primary risk group acquiring AIDS from someone in such a group (such cases are referred to as secondary cases).

The lesson is "unprotected" sexual intercourse presents a risk of HIV transmission, but the greater risks involve homosexual contact and IV drug use. The transmission of HIV requires access to the bloodstream. Clearly, needle sharing provides the necessary access. Sexual transmission is a different issue. In the absence of genital bleeding and lesions, heterosexual sex provides minimal risk of transmission. These facts should not be interpreted to mean that there can be a flippant attitude to the disease. Sexual behavior is still a primary determinant of risk. Abstinence until marriage and fidelity afterwards may be the only form of safe sex around, but a little common sense and knowledge of the facts can go a long way in providing a means of avoiding this disease. Prevention is the only protection (Henderson, 2002).

Hellinger's (1993) estimate for lifetime healthcare costs of treating an AIDS patient was $69,100, a downward revision from its 1992 estimates—it is a trade-off for higher cash wages of $102,000 (CDC, 1999a). The decrease was due to both shorter and less frequent hospital stays. The Food and Drug Administration (FDA) has approved a class of drugs called protease inhibitors which deprive the AIDS virus of a critical enzyme it needs for reproduction. When combined with other older drugs like azidothymidine (AZT) and lamivudine (3TC), this three-drug cocktail suppresses the AIDS virus to undetectable levels (Henderson, 2002).

Now more people can benefit from drug therapy, which is currently priced at $12,000 to $16,000 per person per year. AZT costs $3500 per year, 3TC up to $2800 per year, and the protease inhibitor as high as $7400 per year. Treating all 516,000 HIV-positive and AIDS patients in the United States with combination drug therapy would cost more than $8 billion per year. Adding treatment for an additional 300,000 unreported cases would drive up the cost of treatment to an additional $3 billion, or $5 to $6 billion more than is currently spent. These costs place treatment out of the reach of 90 percent of the world's AIDS sufferers, who live in developing countries (Henderson, 2002).

Although it is estimated that about 40 percent of all AIDS care is financed by government sources, such as Medicaid, the overall impact on the economy is relatively small. Spending on AIDS patients is less than 1 percent of the total healthcare spending in the United States, but it falls disproportionately on public hospitals, especially teaching hospitals in urban areas (Henderson, 2002).

Possibly one of the more disturbing aspects of the AIDS problem is the rebirth of associated diseases that were once considered eradicated in the developed world, such as **tuberculosis (TB)**. A new drug-resistant strain of TB is reappearing among the poor population. The likely cause is the failure of infected people to stick with a regimen of antibiotics for the prescribed treatment periods. In 1953, more than 84,000 cases of TB were reported in the United States. That number fell to 22,255 in 1984. In 1990, TB cases increased 8.4 percent to more than 25,000—the largest single increase since 1953. Since 1993, the number of new cases have fallen every year. By 1999, only 17,531 new cases were reported which was a decrease of almost 30 percent over the previous decade (Henderson, 2002).

Impact Throughout the World

AIDS has reached epidemic proportions in parts of the world. The fastest growing region for HIV infection is Southeast Asia, where 2.5 million already have the disease. In this part of the world, primary transmission of the disease is through heterosexual contact and the male-to-female ratio of those affected stands at about one-to-one. Young adults are the main target of the disease, often with husbands and wives affecting each other. In some areas, adult mortality is doubling or tripling (Henderson, 2002).

The impact has both social and economic components. The disease has left more than 11 million children orphaned. Gaps are also created in the workforce with prime age workers being lost in their most productive years. Life expectancy after contracting AIDS is relatively short in developing countries, primarily due to the lack of funds to care for those affected. More than 95 percent of those with AIDS are in developing countries, but only 6 percent of the money spent on treating the diseases is spent in these countries (Chase, 1992).

The long-term impact of AIDS will be determined by its effect on the labor supply. Fewer workers in the short run due to AIDS-related mortality and fewer births due to the loss of child-bearing females mean fewer workers in the long run. Labor-intensive countries worldwide will see their labor costs rise, increasing the push to less labor-intensive production. This shift is already happening in Africa, where farmers are switching from labor-intensive crops, such as tobacco, to root vegetables which require less labor. A shortage of labor in Africa not only means higher wages in Africa, but ultimately higher wages in the rest of the world. The irony of this epidemic is that even though total economic output may fall for countries that are hardest hit by the disease, per capita output and incomes may rise due to a smaller population (Henderson, 2002).

DRUG ABUSE

Government sources have estimated that approximately 1 in 100 Americans are regular users of cocaine (Kleinman, 1990). Our lack of knowledge on the addictive nature of prolonged use of this drug limits our ability to determine that long-term consequences of regular use, but careful study of the phenomenon clearly shows that drug abuse takes a tremendous toll in terms of human suffering and economic loss to society.

The Extent of Drug Abuse

Overall drug use in the United States has fallen by 50 percent over the years. However, drug use among young adults is rising and fewer teenagers think cocaine is harmful. The 1999 National Household Survey on Drug Use shows:

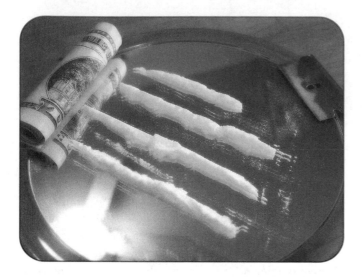

1. Drug use among those aged 12 to 17 increased in 1999 to 10.9 percent. However, for those aged 18 to 25 usage is at its highest level since 1988, increasing to 18.8 percent of that age group. Drug use among adults 26 years old and older has not changed significantly since 1994.

2. Marijuana use doubled from 1992 to 1996. Almost 5 percent of the population aged 12 and older use the drug regularly.

3. In 1999, an estimated 1.5 million Americans were current cocaine users.

4. The monthly use of lysergic acid diethylamide (LSD) and other hallucinogens almost doubled between 1990 and 1998. More than 80 percent of hallucinogens users are under the age of 26.

5. The highest rate of illicit drug use in the United States is found in young adults between the ages 18 to 20 years of age, with rates of current users greater than 20 percent (United States Department of Health and Human Services, 1999).

Despite the overall downward trend, drug use remains a significant American problem.

Healthcare Implications of Cocaine Use

The popularity of cocaine may be attributable to the widespread belief that it is nonaddictive and quite harmless when taken occasionally. This is among the reasons the affect of drug use on hospital emergency rooms across the country. In 1995, serious coronary risk was associated with cocaine use. Numerous studies have shown that the personal health risk associated with the occasional use of cocaine is significant. Anyone suffering from fixed coronary artery disease, and even those who have no previous history of heart disease, assume considerable risk by taking the drug (Henderson, 2002).

Cocaine use causes increased heart rate, elevated systolic blood pressure, and a surge in myocardial oxygen demand. The evidence suggests that the cardiovascular effects of cocaine use include coronary thrombosis and spasms, life-threatening arrhythmias, and in certain cases, rupture of the ascending aorta.

The Drug Abuse Warning Network (DAWN) provides information that adverse effects of cocaine use do not end with acute coronary events. Reasons given to justify its use are mild euphoria, increased alertness, decreased appetite, and enhanced energy. In reality, cocaine is one of the most dangerous drugs in use today. Evidence compiled from animal studies show cocaine to be a powerful reinforcing drug with properties that may lead to compulsive use. The administration of cocaine in recreational doses can result in sleep disorders, assaultive behavior, delirium, nausea, vomiting, chest pain, tremors, seizures, hypertension, hypothermia, respiratory paralysis, cardiac arrhythmias, and even death (Henderson, 2002).

The Drug Abuse Warning Network provides information on the effect of drug use on hospital emergency rooms across the country. In 1995, 531,800 drug-related emergency department episodes were logged in the nation's hospitals. Of that number, 142,500 were cocaine-related, 76,000 were heroin-related, and 47,100 were marijuana-related. Most episodes were connected with a suicide attempt or dependence overdose (SAMHSA, 1996).

Cocaine and Pregnancy

Cocaine use has historically been a phenomenon primarily observed in middle-class males. Today, at least 2 million women use cocaine and crack cocaine. Most of these women are between 20 and 27 years old, the prime child-bearing ages. A recent study by the National Association for Perinatal Addiction Research and Education estimated that at least 8.25 percent and possibly as many as 10 percent of all pregnant women have used cocaine during their pregnancies (Henderson, 2002).

Cocaine has serious effects on birth outcomes. Babies exposed to cocaine in utero have below average birthweights and are more likely to suffer from congenital malformations. In particular, it has been shown that these infants are more likely to have serious gastrointestinal problems and below average head circumferences, resulting in higher than average rates of mental retardation. Cocaine use has serious effects on health (Henderson, 2002).

Even after birth, infants can be exposed to cocaine through their mother's breast milk. The drug will remain in breast milk for up to 60 hours after administration. Even the occasional use by the mother can seriously affect the infant, causing hypertension, rapid heartbeat, sweating, excessive dilation of the pupils, and asphyxiation (Henderson, 2002). Cocaine-exposed infants are also at higher risk for stroke and sudden infant death syndrome.

Cocaine's Cost to Society

Substance abuse is the leading healthcare cost problem in the United States today. Some estimates indicate that more than 60 percent of our healthcare costs are devoted to the treatment of three categories of drugs: alcohol, nicotine, and illegal drugs. The health problems associated with these drugs include heart diseases, emphysema, lung and other cancers, motor vehicle accidents, and birth defects (Henderson, 2002).

Total costs to society of drug abuse runs into the billions of dollars. Drug abuse cost the American society approximately $110 billion per year in 1995 (Harwood et al., 1998). Although this estimate includes the direct and indirect costs of health care, lost productivity, and crime, it fails to adequately measure the emerging healthcare costs for infants exposed to cocaine prenatally, who are referred to as "cocaine babies."

The incidence of maternal drug use is difficult to detect. Drug screening is not a routine procedure in many hospital settings. In any event, recent cocaine use is not always obvious because it does not show up in urine tests until 48 hours after administration. The typical drug-exposed infant will spend 4 to 6 weeks in intensive care after birth. It is not unusual for extremely low birthweight babies to have total hospital bills of at least $100,000. The estimated total cost of intensive care alone for all babies that are affected by drug abuse is over $10.5 billion (Chasnoff et al., 1985).

Intervention Options

The first step in dealing with the drug problem is to establish realistic national goals. For example, is a drug-free America possible? Further, are people willing to change their behaviors?

At the extreme, a great deal of attention has been focused on competing alternatives, namely to legalize and tax drugs that are currently illegal. One advantage of this strategy would be to lower the crime rate by removing the entire genre of criminal acts from the legal code. Opponents argue that, in reality, the people who are committing crimes to support their drug habits are not likely to become model citizens and productive members of society if drug use is legalized.

If economics is to contribute to public policy discussions on this issue, the appropriate questions must be asked. Cost of illness studies are useful in focusing attention on the sheer magnitude of the problem. However, the answer to the complicated questions of optimal allocation of resources will require careful analysis of the effectiveness of individual programs in lowering costs and improving the quality of the lives affected by this national problem (Henderson, 2002).

TOBACCO AND ALCOHOL ABUSE

The health problems associated with alcohol and tobacco use place a serious burden on the United States healthcare sector. Estimating the cost to society requires that the consequences of this behavior be assigned certain economic values. The results of alcohol and tobacco consumption include not only the obvious health problems, such as heart disease, stroke, emphysema, cancer, and cirrhosis of the liver, but also include crime, auto fatalities, and lost productivity on the job.

The estimated cost of alcohol abuse was $166 billion in 1995 (Henderson, 2002). More recent estimates from the CDC place the annual healthcare costs associated with tobacco use between $50 and $73 billion (CDC, 2000). Although the economic costs have been huge, the toll in human suffering cannot place a dollar amount on that reported. It is estimated that more than 100,000 deaths are attributed to alcohol abuse annually. When added to the estimate of 400,000 deaths each year due to tobacco use, the total comes to half a million premature deaths each year from these two substances alone (CDC, 2000).

An overall decline in the prevalence of tobacco use in the United States has occurred among both males and females. Between 1965 and 1998, the average annual rate of decline was 1.5 percent for women and 2.4 percent for men. One disturbing trend is the increased prevalence of tobacco use among high school students. From 1991 to 1999, the percent of high school students who identified themselves as current tobacco users increased from 27.5 percent to 34.8 percent. In fact, 42.8 percent of high school seniors used tobacco in 1999. Overall, the prevalence of tobacco use by gender differs between 3 to 5 percentage points for most age groups. However, among high school students, the prevalence of use between boys and girls differs little (MMWR, 2000).

One of the reasons that women live longer in most societies is that they do not smoke with the same regularity as men. Even so, more than 500,000 women are dying worldwide every year of smoking-related illnesses. By the time today's young female population reaches middle age, more than 1 million females will be dying annually from smoking-related illness in the developed world alone (Henderson, 2002).

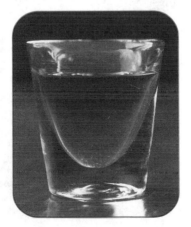

SOCIAL PROBLEMS

Many of the social problems we face in the United States find their way to the emergency departments and trauma wards of the nation's hospitals. Substance abuse [discussed in prior section], violence, and sexual promiscuity [discussed in prior section] lead the total number of health problems that our healthcare sector must deal with on a daily basis. Other issues include teen pregnancy, sexually transmitted diseases and homelessness, which are addressed below.

Violence

Violent crimes in the United States totaled 1,430,693 in 1999, down more than 25 percent from 1992 levels. This number includes 15,533 murders, 89,107 forcible rapes, and 916,383 aggravated assaults (U.S. Department of Justice, 1999). The male per capita homicide rate in the United States is 10 to 12 times that experienced in Britain and Germany and 5 times the rate in Canada (Schwartz, 1991). Death rates in the United States vary considerably by ethnic group. The leading cause of death for blacks between the ages of 15 and 24 is homicide. The homicide rate for black males in that age category is nine times the rate of that for white males. HIV is the leading cause of death for black males between 25 and 44 years of age. For whites in these two age categories, accidents cause more deaths than any other cause (Singh et al., 1996).

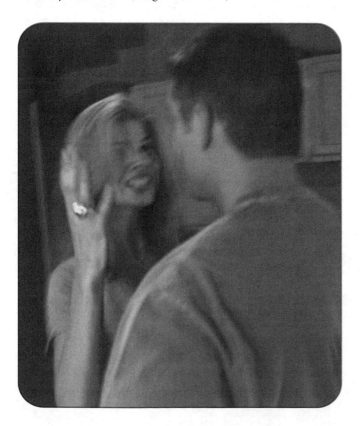

Virtually every homicide and forcible rape results in an emergency department visit. Also, United States emergency departments report 100 assaults for every homicide visit. But of all the tragic consequences of criminal violence, the most perplexing problem facing many poor inner-city neighborhoods is domestic violence. Although it is not confined to the inner city or any particular ethnic group, this problem seems to manifest itself and grow in a culture and philosophy that thrives in the inner city (Henderson, 2002). Assault by a male partner is the leading cause of emergency department visits for women (McKibben et al., 1989). The facts include:

1. In an average 12-month period, two million American women are severely beaten by their male partners.
2. More than half of the women murdered in the United States are killed by a current or former male partner.
3. Twenty percent of all adult women, 15 percent of all college women, and 12 percent of adolescent girls will experience sexual abuse or assault in their lifetimes.
4. More than one-third of all obstetric patients are abused while they are pregnant. (Browne, 1992)

Whatever the causes of domestic violence, a greater acceptance of its use to settle disputes seems prevalent in our society. Whether it is traced to the decline in family values or whether it is the product of government neglect, domestic violence is an issue that is eating away at the moral fabric of our society. If this deterioration continues, no amount of spending in health care will be able to reconstruct the broken lives and rectify intense human suffering it causes.

Teen Pregnancy

Teen pregnancy and illegitimacy may actually serve as proxy variables for maternal behavior and attitude about pregnancy (Pamuk and Mosher, 1988). Teen mothers are more likely to receive inadequate prenatal care, smoke cigarettes, have infants with low birthweights, and experience a higher rate of preterm births (Ventura et al., 2000). One report based on data from the National Center for Health Statistics indicated that unmarried college students have higher infant mortality rates than married women, regardless of their educational attainment (Eberstadt, 1991).

Births to teenage and unmarried women in the United States are declining in almost all racial and ethnic categories. The teenage pregnancy rate fell 17.7 percent between 1991 and 1998. The black and Hispanic rates have fallen to 85.4 per 1000 teenage females and 93.6 per 1000 females, respectively, but are still approximately twice the rate of whites at 45.4 per 1000. Although the overall rate of teenage births has been declining since 1991, the proportion of births to unmarried teenagers rose to 78.9 percent in 1998. Even with this high rate of illegitimacy among teenage mothers, more than 70 percent of the births to unmarried women are to mothers over the age of 20 (Henderson, 2002).

Limited access to prenatal care due to limited finances, while often cited as a factor of low birthweights, may not be the primary cause. In the District of Columbia, where prenatal care is provided free of charge at 11 of the city's 16 health clinics, the infant mortality rate is the nation's worst, at 27 per 1000 in 1989 (Singh, 1990). Adjusting for the mother's age, education, and other characteristics related to risk, black mothers were more likely to forego prenatal care completely, to begin prenatal care later than their white counterparts, and to have fewer prenatal physician visits. When they did take advantage of medical benefits, black mothers still had twice the rate of low birthweight babies than whites (Murray and Bernfield, 1988).

Low birthweights lead to longer hospital stays, driving up the cost of newborn care. Normal sized infants (weighing more than 2500 grams) can expect to stay in the hospital up to 3 days. Smaller infants, those weighing between 1500 and 2500 grams, have average stays of 24 days. Those born weighing less than 1500 grams have average stays of 57 days and those less than 1000 grams have average stays of 89 days (McCormick, 1985).

International comparisons are frequently made to stimulate policy discussion, but the comparisons should be made with caution due to variation in measurement issues across countries. Infant mortality and teen pregnancy issues are important health problems. For a number of reasons, the United States rankings on these dimensions are relatively low (Henderson, 2002).

Sexually Transmitted Disease

Sexual promiscuity is undermining the public health of the nation. Unwise sexual practices, such as first intercourse at an early age, multiple sex partners, and high frequency of intercourse have led to an epidemic of **sexually transmitted diseases (STDs)**. The CDC estimates that 65 million Americans have an incurable STD, and most are infected with genital herpes. More than 15 million new cases are diagnosed each year with two-thirds of those diagnosed being younger than 25 years of age. Cases of syphilis and gonorrhea are at all-time lows, but others, such as genital herpes and chlamydia continue to spread at alarming rates (CDC, 1999b). Except for the common cold or flu, STDs are the most common diseases in North America (CDC, 1993a and 1993b).

A study released by the CDC in 1997 reported that 1.2 million adolescents or 5.6 percent of the 12 to 19 year-old population is infected with genital herpes. The CDC alone spends in excess of $100 million annually for treatment and prevention of syphilis, gonorrhea, chlamydia, and herpes with little to show for

it. Active herpes sores open up a pathway to the bloodstream, making those with open lesions ten times more likely to acquire HIV than those without such lesions (Peterson, 1997).

The human papillomavirus (HPV) is the most common STD among young sexually active populations. A recent study (Ho et al., 1998) found that approximately 14 percent of all women attending college are infected with HPV each year. More than 40 percent of the women in the study were infected with HPV during the 3-year period. HPV is particularly troublesome because most people who suffer from it are asymptomatic and it can lead to cervical, penile, and anal cancer.

Another growing problem is the number of women of reproductive age suffering from *Chlamydia trachomatis*. Chlamydia infections are common among sexually active adolescents and young people, numbering over 4 million per year. Asymptomatic in most women, if untreated it leads to pelvic inflammatory disease (PID). PID is an infection of the upper reproductive tract caused primarily by sexually transmitted organisms. More than 2.5 million new cases of PID are reported annually, affecting 10 to 15 percent of all reproductive-age women during their lifetimes. More than 250,000 women are hospitalized annually and more than 100,000 surgeries are performed due to PID (Henderson, 20002).

The efficacy of condom use on the incidence of STDs is widely debated. One group believes that the distribution and widespread use of condoms will reduce the spread of sexually transmitted diseases and teenage pregnancy. The other group argues that easy access to condoms actually exacerbates the problems by encouraging dangerous sexual practices. With little hard evidence to support either set of claims, the United States experiences occurrences of STD infection among adolescents aged 15 to 19 at alarming figures (Henderson, 2002).

Homelessness

The homeless population in the United States has been estimated at somewhere between 250,000 and 3 million. The extreme variation in the estimates is due to the absence of a uniform definition of homelessness (Henderson, 2002).

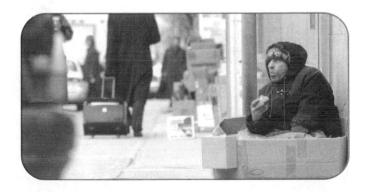

Regardless of which definition is used, homelessness is associated with a range of social, mental health, criminal, alcohol, and drug problems. The United States homeless population is 75 percent male. The majority is white, but blacks and Native Americans are disproportionately represented. Most are isolated from family through divorce, widowhood, or being never married. Those still living in family units are almost exclusively female (Rossi et al., 1987).

The homeless suffer from a wide range of physical and mental health problems. Alcohol and drug abuse is common. Severe depression, suicide, psychotic symptoms, and previous psychiatric hospitalizations are common. In addition, there is a high incidence of contact with the criminal justice system, often for alcohol and drug-related reasons and characteristics. These physical and mental disabilities, coupled with the extreme poverty experienced by most of the homeless, complicates our task of dealing with the problem (Henderson, 2002).

SUMMARY

In this chapter, a number of socioeconomic concerns have been addressed that affect the overall health of the population. Alcohol, drug, and tobacco use and their associated health problems increase the demand for health care and are responsible for a large percentage of overall healthcare spending in this nation. Teen pregnancy, illegitimacy, domestic violence, STDs, and homelessness are experienced at higher levels in the United States than in other developed countries in the world.

The government's role is not limited to legislative options. Subsidy and tax options can also serve to encourage healthy behavior and discourage unhealthy behavior. The challenges are enormous and suggest that economics can play a role in those sensitive areas of public policymaking.

Key Words

■ Acquired immunodeficiency syndrome (AIDS)

■ Tuberculosis (TB)

■ Sexually transmitted disease (STD)

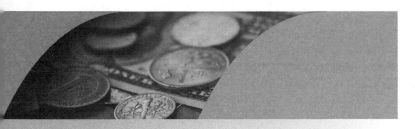

Questions

1. How important is the deterioration of the social system in contributing to the healthcare spending crisis?

2. Is it important to characterize such social problems as alcoholism and drug abuse as diseases rather than behavior disorders?

3. What are the implications for the healthcare system with the proliferation of new diseases?

4. The best way to lower the incidence of STDs is to make condoms widely available to teenagers and educate them on their proper use. Do you agree or disagree? Explain.

REFERENCES

1. Browne, A. (1992) Violence against women: relevance for medical practitioners. *Journal of the American Medical Association,* 254(1):81–83.

2. Centers for Disease Control and Prevention. (2000) Youth tobacco surveillance—United States 1998–1999. *Morbidity and Mortality Weekly Report, Surveillance Summary,* 49(SS10):1–93.

3. ———— (1999a) *HIV/AIDS Surveillance Report,* 11(2).

4. ———— (1999b) *Tracking the Hidden Epidemics: Trends in the STD Epidemics in the United States.*

5. ———— (1993a) Recommendations for the prevention and management of Chlamydia trachomatis infections, 1993. *Morbidity and Mortality Weekly Report,* Recommendations and Reports, 42, No. RR–12.

6. ———— (1993b) 1993 sexually transmitted disease treatment guidelines. *Morbidity and Mortality Weekly Reports,* 42, No. RR–14.

7. Chase, M. (1992). Researcher sees U.S. cost of treating AIDS virus rising sharply by 1995. *Wall Street Journal,* July 23:B8.

8. Chasnoff, IJ et al. (1985) Cocaine use in pregnancy. *New England Journal of Medicine,* 313(11):666–669.

9. Eberstadt, N. (1991) American's infant-mortality puzzle. *The Public Interest,* 105:30–47.

10. Harwood, H et al. (1998) *The economic costs of alcohol and drug abuse in the United States, 1992.* National Institutes of Health, Publication No. 98–4327.

11. Hellinger, FJ. (1993) The lifetime costs of treating a person with HIV. *Journal of the American Medical Association,* 270(4):474–478.

12. Henderson, JW. (2002) *Health Economics and Policy,* 2d ed. Mason, Ohio: South-Western.

13. Ho, GYF et al. (1998) Natural history of cervicovaginal papillomavirus infection in young women. *New England Journal of Medicine,* 388(7):423–428.

14. Holmberg, S. (1996) The estimated prevalence and incidence of HIV in 96 large U.S. metropolitan areas. *American Journal of Public Health,* 86(5):642–654.

15. Kleinman, MAR. (1990) *Hard core cocaine addicts: measuring—and fighting—the epidemic.* A staff report prepared for the use of the Committee on the Judiciary, U.S. Senate. Washington DC: U.S. Government Printing Office, 105–118.

16. McCormick, MC. (1985) The contribution of low birthweight to infant mortality and childhood morbidity. *New England Journal of Medicine,* 312(2):82–90.

17. McKibben, L. deVoss, E, and EH Newberger. (1989) Victimization of mothers of abused children: a controlled study. *Pediatrics,* 84(9):531–535.

18. MMWR. (2000) Guidelines for preventing opportunistic infections among stem cell transplant recipients. *MMWR,* October 20, 2000; 49:1–128.

19. Murray, JL and M Bernfield. (1988) The differential effect of prenatal care on the incidence of low birthweight among blacks and whites in a prepaid health care plan. *New England Journal of Medicine,* 319(21):1385–1390.

20. Pamuk, ER and WD Mosher. (1988) *Health Aspects of Pregnancy and Childbirth: United States, 1982.* Hyattsville, MD: National Center for Health Statistics.

21. Peterson, A. (1997) Overshadowed by AIDS, herpes spreads alarmingly. *Wall Street Journal,* December 10:B1, B12.

22. Rossi, PH et al. (1987) The urban homeless: estimating composition and size. *Science,* 28:1336–1341.

23. Schwartz, L. (1991) The medical costs of America's social ills. *Wall Street Journal,* June 24:A12.

24. Singh, GK, Kochanek, KD and MF MacDorman. (1996) Advance report of final mortality statistics, 1994. *Monthly Vital Statistics Report,* 45(3) Supplement. Centers for Disease Control and Prevention.

25. Singh, HKD. (1990) Stork reality: why America's infants are dying. *Policy Review,* 56–63.

26. Substance Abuse and Mental Health Services Administration (SAMHSA). (1996) National drug survey results released. SAMHSA Press Release, August 20.

27. U.S. Department of Justice (1999). *Crime in the United States, 1999: Uniform Crime Reports.* Washington, DC: Federal Bureau of Investigation.

28. Ventura, SJ, Curtin SC, and TJ Mathews. (2000). Variations in teenage birth rates, 1991–1998: national and state trends. *National Vital Statistics Reports*, 48(6). Hyattsville, MD: National Center for Health Statistics.

BIO: ALAIN ENTHOVEN

Alain Enthoven is a leading figure in the healthcare reform movement. His ideas have helped shape recent reforms in England and the Netherlands. It was also Enthoven who served as the intellectual backbone of the famous "Jackson Hole Group" that has regularly studied and discussed healthcare reform since the mid-1970s. A respected Stanford Economist, Enthoven is a strong proponent of managed competition.

After completing his undergraduate work at Stanford, he received a Rhodes scholarship to study at Oxford. In 1956, he completed his PhD in economics from MIT and went to work for the RAND Corporation in Santa Monica, California. His early work was on defense issues, and he soon became knowledgeable in the ways of the federal government. He became well known in governmental circles and went to work at the Pentagon in 1961. During his years in Washington, he became a director of Georgetown University. While on the board, he was chairman of the committee that built a major medical center at the school and created the university's group practice health maintenance organization (HMO).

In 1973, Enthoven began consulting at the Kaiser-Permanente Group in California, where he developed most of his ideas for reforming medical care. That same year, he joined the Stanford faculty where he is now the Marriner S. Eccles Professor of Public and Private Management in the Graduate School of Business and Professor of Health Research in the School of Medicine.

Enthoven (1988) argued that "reform should start with cost-conscious choices made by the educated middle class. In this way, the organizational cultures of health plans are created in an environment in which they serve intelligent, relatively informed people who have choices."

Source: John Huber. "The Abandoned Father of Health Care Reform," *The New York Times Magazine*, July 18, 1993, 24–26, 36–37.

Health Economics and Policy, 2nd Edition. James W. Henderson. (Cincinnati, OH: South-western, 2002).

The Hospital Industry

THE FLEXNOR REPORT

The publication of the Flexnor Report in 1910 served as a catalyst for general reform in healthcare delivery. This report was a critical review of medical education in the United States. The response of the medical establishment led to changes in the accreditation processes of medical schools and an improvement in the quality of medical care. Nowhere are the effects more noticeable than in the hospital industry. Hospitals, once notorious places more likely to spread disease than cure them, have since been transformed into the focal point of the medical care delivery system (Johnson-Lans, 2004).

This chapter examines the market for hospital services. The first two sections provide a brief history of hospitals and an examination of the institutional setting in the United States. They are followed by a discussion of the role of the private, not-for-profit hospitals as the dominant organization in the industry. This chapter also examines popular theories of hospital behavior and finally, recent developments in the industry, in particular the trend toward multihospital systems.

A BRIEF HISTORY OF AMERICAN HOSPTIALS

Drawing on Stevens' work (1989), three important factors served to transform hospitals into the modern medical institutions they have become today: the germ theory of disease, advances in medical technology, and increased urbanization. These changes have been accompanied by a dramatic change in patient expectations. No longer do patients seek a caring environment exclusively, they have come to expect a cure.

The development of the germ theory of disease, first articulated by Louis Pasteur in 1870, revolutionized the treatment of diseases. Diseases were seen as having specific causes, rather than merely viewing them as a disequilibrium. The search for causal factors required more elaborate testing and diagnostic services. Centralized medical care, bringing the patient to the practitioner, became a necessity (Johnson-Lans, 2004).

Now, hospital technology—especially advances in surgical and diagnostic imaging—provided physicians with the tools that would revolutionize medical intervention. Anesthesia was first used in surgery in 1846. But it was not until the adoption of antiseptic procedures, beginning in 1867, that the high rates of death from infection following surgery began to fall. The introduction of X-ray technology in the late 1800s, and more recently, the development of more advanced imaging (e.g., CT scans and MRIs) vastly improved the ability to diagnose injury and illness (Johnson-Lans, 2004).

A third factor, urbanization, also played an important role in the centralization of medical facilities. Migration to urban centers meant more one-person households and fewer extended families living together. People could no longer count on treatment at home. Home was an apartment or boarding house and likely inappropriate for convalescence. Without family nearby, patients had no one to serve as caregivers (Johnson-Lans, 2004).

When hospitals were financed through taxation and philanthropy, patient fees were only of minor importance. As middle-class use of hospital services increased, changes in financing were inevitable. By 1900, patients' fees comprised more than one-third of hospital income (Johnson-Lans, 2004).

What has become to be known as the modern hospital began to emerge in the twentieth century. The important developments that led to today's acute care facility are summarized here (Johnson-Lans, 2004):

1900–1915: The Flexnor Report (1910) served as a pointed condemnation of medical education. In its wake, bogus medical schools were closed, standards became more stringent, and the goal of scientific medicine was employed. The general reform of medicine led to affiliations between medical schools and hospitals and ultimately the formulation of the teaching hospital.

1920s: Continued reforms were aimed at driving incompetent physicians out of the profession. Physician licensing became more structured and hospital admission privileges were restricted to members of certain medical societies. The decade also saw the role of nurses change dramatically. Prior to the 1928 nursing reforms, poorly-trained volunteers or nurses in training did most of the nursing in the hospital. Trained nurses established community practices that directly competed with hospitals. After the reforms, nurses no longer competed with hospitals.

1930s: The reliance on patient fees caused severe financial problems for hospitals during the Great Depression. The introduction of private health insurance during the decade would transform medical care financing. Modeled after a prepaid hospital plan for Dallas schoolteachers developed by Baylor University Hospital, the American Hospital Association (AHA) established the first Blue Cross plan and soon had a monopoly in hospital insurance.

The decade also saw a revolution in pharmaceuticals. The most important advance was the development of sulfa drugs and penicillin. For the first time, physicians had the power to cure diseases based on infection.

1940s: Wartime demands resulted in a sharp increase in the number of physicians and nurses in training. The war provided a unique opportunity to improve skills and develop new techniques. The federal government also became actively involved in providing hospital care. The passage of the Hill-Burton Act in 1946 dedicated the government to replacing the aging hospital infrastructure that had deteriorated during the Depression and war. With priority given to hospital construction in rural or poor areas of the country, Hill-Burton served

to create a climate in the hospital sector making uncompensated care an expected element of the overall healthcare financing mechanism.

Precluded from offering higher wages because of rigid price controls, companies were forced to compete for workers by offering better benefits packages, including employer-provided health insurance. A ruling by the National Labor Relations Board in 1948 made health insurance a permanent feature in labor negotiations by ruling that it was subject to collective bargaining. Tax deductible for the employer and tax exempt for the employee, group health plans now cover more than one-half of all workers with private health insurance.

1950s: Vaccines against polio and rubella marked the true beginning of high technology medicine. These developments, combined with the widespread use of antibiotics, helped change the image of medicine. Physicians were no longer practitioners with limited knowledge able only to ease suffering. Patients now expected to leave the doctor's office cured. The anticipated number of doctor and hospital visits during a person's lifetime increased significantly, along with the concern over how to pay for them. The result was an increased demand for private health insurance.

Advances in medical research tools highlighted the decade. The light microscope with magnification of 2000 times had been in use since the 17th century. The development of the electron microscope with magnification of one million times allowed the study of cell structure and metabolism.

1960s: Congress created Medicare and Medicaid, making the federal government the major purchaser of healthcare services. Physicians who opposed the program as "socialized medicine" and prophesied ruin under a government-run system, soon learned to love it. No longer worried about the ability of the elderly and the indigent to pay their doctor bills, physicians' earnings rose rapidly. Today, more than half of physicians' income comes from government sources.

The decade also witnessed the beginnings of the investor-owned, for-profit hospital system. Prior to the mid 1960s, for-profit hospitals were small, rare, and established to benefit clearly defined patient groups. Until the creation of Medicare and Medicaid, the general population with large numbers of elderly and uninsured was not a dependable source of revenue. Therefore, Medicare and Medicaid, serving as a stable funding source, actually facilitated the development of the for-profit hospital sector.

1970s: Explosive growth typified the medical care system. New hospitals and clinics, medical school admissions, foreign-educated doctors, open heart surgery, transplants, and helicopter ambulances were widespread. The total number of surgeries increased from 14.8 million in 1972 to 24.6 million in 1997. Much of the increase was necessary. Nevertheless, it was an ominous sign when the procedures most lucrative to physicians under the payment system in place escalated at the fastest rate.

The intensity of medical interventions also increased dramatically. Intensive care units (ICUs) became widely used. Trauma centers were established in most areas. Although the trauma center is one of those expenses that may be worth the cost, the ICU in contrast, has created a painful dilemma. Originally designed for temporary use following surgery or shock, its function has been extended to the terminally ill who have little likelihood of recovery.

All the developments of the 1970s shared one thing in common: they were all expensive. Healthcare expenditures increased at a rate of 13 percent yearly. By the end of the decade, Medicare expenditures were growing at an annual rate of 20 percent annually. Concerned over the spending growth, state rate-setting legislation and certificate of need (CON) laws were used more frequently. CON laws required governmental approval for capital expansion projects in hospitals, including bed capacity and medical equipment. In practice, CON laws served to reduce competition and actually limited the entry of HMOs and nursing homes in some markets (Mayo and McFarland, 1989).

1980s: By 1982, healthcare expenditures exceeded 10 percent of gross domestic product for the first time. To slow the rate of growth in federal expenditures, Medicare initiated a new hospital reimbursement method based on the diagnosis, rather than the services performed. Implemented in 1983, diagnosis-related groups (DRGs) have had profound effects on the hospital industry, moving a large percentage of the financing from retrospective to prospective payment.

1990s: Managed care has been the dominant factor affecting medical care delivery during this decade. Capitation and risk sharing have transformed the industry. Hospitals are no longer the revenue generators they once were, but instead they have become cost centers. **Horizontal integration**—characterized by hospital mergers and consolidations—transformed an industry once highly fragmented with many stand-alone facilities, into one where multihospital systems are common. A system characterized by underutilization and overstaffing now experiences a move toward integrated systems and a wave of not-for-profit to for-profit conversions. With administrators downsizing in the name of **efficiency**, many critics wonder about issues of quality of care and the provision of indigent care.

THE U.S. INSTITUTIONAL SETTING

Hospitals are by far the most important institutional setting for the provision of medical services. In 1999, hospital expendi-

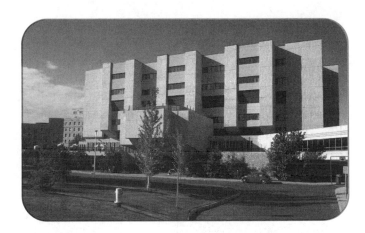

tures totaled more than $390 billion, which is one-third the national healthcare spending, and more than 4 percent of gross domestic product. In addition to high overall spending, the hospital is also the most expensive setting on a per-unit basis. (Johnson-Lans, 2004)

Hospital Classification

Hospitals are classified according to the length of stay, the major type of service delivered, and the type of ownership. Hospitals with average lengths of stay of less than 30 days are classified as short-term hospitals. Long-term hospitals are those with an average length of stay of over 30 days.

Community Hospitals

Community hospitals are the most common hospital classified by types of services offered. Under the current classification method adopted in 1972, a community hospital is defined as a short-stay hospital, providing not only general services, but also specialty care, including obstetrics and gynecology; eye, ear, nose, and throat; and rehabilitation and orthopedic services. Other hospitals are classified according to specialized services offered. They include hospitals that provide psychiatric services and hospitals that treat individuals with tuberculosis and other respiratory diseases.

Drawing from Henderson (2002), community hospitals are also classified according to control or ownership. The most prominent form of ownership is the private not-for-profit hospital, representing 60 percent of all hospitals. For-profit hospitals represent 15.4 percent of all community hospitals and 13.4 percent of all beds. The remaining 24.6 percent of community hospitals are government owned, usually by the states. Community hospital figures do not include approximately 285 federal hospitals with almost 62,000 beds.

More than 85 percent of all nonfederal hospitals are classified as community hospitals. The number of community hospitals peaked in the early 1980s. Since then, the decline has been about 1 percent per year, until 1998 when the number stood at 5015. Most of the decline has come from small and rural hospitals, many of which had been government owned. The number of beds experienced a similar downward trend. Until the mid 1980s, the number of beds declined faster than the number of hospitals. The number of beds per 1000 population stood at 4.38 in 1980. The steady decline since then left the United States with 3.11 beds per 1000 in 1998. Despite the number of hospitals declining, the number of beds falling, and physicians admitting fewer patients, the average occupancy rates have also fallen dramatically. In 1980, on average more than three-fourths of the beds were occupied. By 1990, that fraction had fallen to barely two-thirds and by 1998 it stood at 62.5 percent.

Even as the number of hospitals has decreased, the number of freestanding ambulatory care centers has increased dramatically, including surgical centers, physical therapy centers, and diagnostic imaging centers, many of which are owned and operated by physicians. Competing directly with hospitals, these facilities may have a competitive advantage because both rely on referrals from physicians for their patients. Government policy and professional ethics serve to reduce any conflict of interest by placing restrictions on self-referral to physician-owned facilities.

Teaching Hospitals

About 20 percent of all hospitals in the United States have an affiliation with one or more of the nation's 125 medical schools and sponsor at least one residency training program. More than 400 hospitals belong to the Council of Teaching Hospitals of the Association of American Medical Colleges. To qualify for membership in this association, a hospital must participate in at least four approved residency programs. Nationwide, 80 of these teaching hospitals are university owned and 70 are operated by the Department of Veterans Affairs (AAMC, 1999).

Most of the teaching hospitals are located in major metropolitan areas with populations in excess of one million. On average, they have more beds, longer patient stays, and higher occupancy rates than their nonteaching counterparts with predictable results—higher costs. Not only are teaching and research expensive, but because of a significant presence in the inner-city, these hospitals find their emergency rooms and outpatient clinics filled with uninsured patients seeking free care.

Recognizing the legitimacy of these higher costs of education and research, federal government provides subsidies, both direct and indirect, to supplement hospital revenues. Direct subsidies include stipends for residents, salaries for teaching physicians, grants for research, and overhead payments for administrative expenses. Indirect subsidies are provided in the form of higher reimbursement rates for Medicare patients. With cutbacks in Medicare reimbursements, teaching hospitals are finding that they too must respond to the prospects of a more competitive market place (Johnson-Lans, 2004).

Hospital Spending

The growth in the hospital sector can be seen more clearly upon examining the change in expenses (excluding new construction) for community hospitals and the total hospital sector. Hospital spending has increased from $9.3 billion in 1960 to $390 billion in 1999. The average growth rates in hospital spending were well over 10 percent per year through much of the 1980s. Spending has abated somewhat, increasing at less than 4 percent per year since 1994 (Henderson, 2002). The moderation in spending growth may be in part attributable to the introduction of prospective payment in 1983. Hospital spending had increased to almost 40 percent of total healthcare expenditures since 1985. Since that time, hospital spending has fallen to 32 percent of total healthcare expenditures (Henderson, 2002).

Most hospital spending is by third party payers. Government sources pay more than 60 percent of all spending, with Medicare and Medicaid providing approximately three-fourths of that amount. Private insurance pays about 30 percent. Patients pay 3.4 percent out-of-pocket and the remaining 5 percent is paid from private funds, primarily charity donations and miscellaneous hospital revenues (e.g., gift shops, parking, and cafeterias). The patient share of hospital spending, 3 cents out of every $1, has fallen over the past 40 years from almost 21 cents in 1960 (Henderson, 2002).

Because Medicare and Medicaid costs comprise such a large percentage of the total hospital bill, government reimbursement rules play a big role in determining the financial stability of the hospital sector. Pressure from Congress to slow the rate of spending has contributed to a complicated system of subsidies and cross-subsidies among payers. Morrisey (1995) reported that Medicare paid 85 percent of the actual costs incurred by hospitals in 1992 and Medicaid paid 78 percent. In addition to these underpayments, hospitals provided billions of dollars in uncompensated care to the uninsured. To make up the shortfall, patients covered by private insurance were charged 138 percent of actual costs incurred in treating them, a practice called cost shifting.

Structure of the Hospital Market

Economics predicts that competition in most markets improves economic welfare. This improvement in economic welfare comes as a result of lower prices, improved efficiency, and higher quality. But does this prediction hold in the hospital sector? Before answering this question, an exploration of how competitive the hospital sector is in the first place is in order.

Competition may be viewed from the perspective of how well a market fits the characteristics of the perfectly competitive model. Applying the discussion from an earlier chapter, competition depends on the number of firms in the market, the nature of the product offered, the relative ease of entering the market with a competing firm, and the amount of information available to consumers.

Hospital markets may not fit the competitive model very well because so many of the structural characteristics of perfect competition are violated. Local markets, where most hospital services are purchased, typically have a limited number of hospitals. Services are not standardized across hospitals. In fact, hospitals expend a considerable amount of resources to differentiate themselves from their rivals. Relatively uninformed consumers who, for the most part, leave the decision making to their physicians, characterize the decision-making process. Third party insurance pays for most of the care, leaving patients insensitive to price differences (Henderson, 2002).

No theoretical basis is available for determining the minimum number of hospitals needed to sustain a competitive environment. How many providers are needed to promote competition? In many metropolitan areas, numerous hospitals provide a complete range of medical services, conveniently located within a short distance of perhaps several hundred thousand residents. For example, the Dallas-Fort Worth metroplex with a population of 4.86 million in 1998 had 70 hospitals, most located within a reasonable commute of one another. In fact, approximately 42 percent of the population of the United States lives in metropolitan areas with more than 1.2 million inhabitants. Based on the number of hospitals per 1000 inhabitants nationwide, a metropolitan area of this size would have approximately 23 hospitals. In 1990, more than 70 percent of the population lived in markets with more than 180,000 inhabitants, a minimum size necessary to provide a full range of acute care hospital services to the surrounding community (Henderson, 2002). An area this size could likely support three or four community hospitals. The fact that physicians make most of the important decisions regarding hospital care may be a problem if demand inducement can be shown to be an extensive problem.

Several attempts have been made to examine the issue of hospital competition empirically. Held and Pauly (1983) found little evidence of price competition among hospitals. They do seem to compete, but competition is based on quality of care and other amenities, not price. Robinson et al. (1988) could only find competition on certain nonprice aspects of the hospital stay, where longer stays occur in regions that have more

hospitals. Following this line of reasoning, research seems to indicate that as competition increases in the hospital sector, costs tend to increase (Luft et al., 1986; Robinson and Luft, 1987).

Feldman and Dowd (1986) approached the question from a different perspective. They suggested that the answer to the question could be determined by estimating the price elasticity of demand for individual hospitals. Price elasticities close to infinity (or at least significantly greater than one) would provide evidence for competitive markets. Using data from the early 1980s, they concluded that certain patient groups, especially Medicare patients, had no price sensitivity at all. Thus, hospital markets did not seem to be competitive.

Although early empirical evidence does not seem to support the hypothesis that hospital markets are competitive, the research was conducted prior to the recent expansion of managed care as a way of organizing and financing medical care delivery. The use of DRGs began to put pressure on hospitals in the mid 1980s to limit the use of nonprice competitive strategies that had been so prevalent. The expanded use of prospective payment in managed care also resulted in more price competition. The relationship between payer and provider is changing dramatically, characterized by aggressive negotiations over prices. Some hospital markets may be more competitive than others, but all are experiencing increased competition (Henderson, 2002).

The best evidence at this time leads us to conclude that competition in the hospital sector during the 1980s did result in a medical arms race that improved the quality of care for some patients, but also drove up costs substantially (Kessler and McClellan, 2000; Keeler et al., 1999). Furthermore, as competition continued to escalate in the 1990s, quality began to improve and costs began to fall in spite of increased concentration, supporting the predictions of traditional economic analysis.

THE ROLE OF THE NOT-FOR-PROFIT ORGANIZATION IN THE HOSPITAL INDUSTRY

At the turn of the 20th century, most hospitals were organized as not-for-profit institutions. Their main responsibility was the provision of free care for the poor and indigent. Hospitals were notorious institutions—avoided at all costs by self-respecting people. Medical reform during the pre-war years enhanced the quality and respectability of hospitals. Paying customers provided the incentive for the development of the proprietary for-profit institution. The financial challenges of the Great Depression and government policy favoring the not-for-profit structure led to the dominance of the private, not-for-profit hospital after the Second World War. With their tax-exempt status, not-for-profit hospitals were able to accept tax deductible charitable contributions. Many received construction subsidies from the federal government under the Hill-Burton Act. Some state legislatures even made the for-profit form illegal altogether. As a result by 1998, more than three-fourths of all community hospitals were either government-owned or not-for-profit (Henderson, 2002).

The Not-For-Profit Organizational Form

Substantial differences can be seen in the institutional constraints facing for-profit and not-for-profit hospitals. For all practical purposes, the differences can be summarized as differences in the right to transfer assets. A not-for-profit hospital does not have shareholders in the typical sense of the term. Thus, equity capital does not come from the sale of stock, but from donations. Without shares of stock, no dividends are paid. Surplus funds are restricted and may not be used to provide ex post incentives to managers. In other words, hospital administrators may not receive dividends or other distributions of residual earnings at the end of the accounting period. Finally, in the event of liquidation or sale of assets, no individual owners receive the proceeds (Henderson, 2002).

Only recently have economists begun to examine the incentive structure facing not-for-profit managers. Influential research by Alchian and Densetz (1972) contrasted the incentives facing for-profit and not-for-profit managers. Pauly (1987) extended the thinking by noting that all successful enterprises generate surplus income. Not-for-profit managers, unable to extract the surplus for themselves in the form of profit-sharing, will extract it in nonpecuniary forms.

Nature of Competition in the Not-For-Profit Sector

The popularity of the not-for-profit organizational form in the hospital industry may seem a bit odd given the dominance of the for-profit firm in the rest of the United States economy. Sloan (1988) addresses the conventional wisdom regarding the prevalence of not-for-profit hospitals. The first argument is based on asymmetric information in the hospital market. Because patients have a difficult time evaluating the quality of health care, they prefer to purchase their health care from providers who do not suffer from the profit motive. If this assumption is true, however, no good reason explains why virtually every other provider—physicians, optometrists, pharmacists, and dentists—works for the for-profit sector (Henderson, 2002).

A second argument is based on the notion that profit-maximizing hospitals will not undertake any activity where the marginal revenue is less than the marginal costs. Activities such as biomedical research, medical education, and public health would not be provided at optimal levels. In addition, patients

without insurance or other means of paying would be less likely to receive care. This line of reasoning, while relevant for teaching and large public hospitals, cannot explain why the rest of the not-for-profit sector engages in little research, undertakes few public health activities, and provides no more uncompensated care than hospitals in the for-profit sector (Sloan et al. , 1986).

Based on arguments by Pauly and Redisch (1973) and Shalit (1977), hospitals are not-for-profit because this form of organization provides the most benefits for physicians. Patients do not purchase hospital services directly. Their physician-agents do it for them. Hospitals, rather than competing for patients, actually compete for physicians, who admit patients. Physicians, interested in maximizing their own productivity, will have more control over decisions relating to the input mix in the absence of the profit motive.

Many argue that even with the preponderance of not-for-profits in the industry, the profit-maximizing objective is a reasonable operating assumption. Operating margins (operating revenues less operating expenses) are positive for most hospitals, even the not-for-profit ones. This operating surplus has many uses. It can be used to increase the incomes of staff physicians or other personnel or it can be used to promote desired activities, such as teaching and research. To the extent that hospitals are run to further the interests of physicians, financial and otherwise, the use of the profit-maximizing model may be reasonable (Henderson, 2002).

Thus, decision making in a not-for-profit hospital resembles decision making in a for-profit hospital (Danzon, 1982). With free entry and free exit in the hospital sector, Newhouse (1970) notes that all hospitals, for-profit and not-for-profit, must produce efficiently to survive. The empirical evidence is far from unanimous on the issue. Zelder (1999) reviewed 24 studies comparing for-profit and not-for-profit performance in the hospital sector. One-half of the studies found no significant difference in operating behavior between the two organizational forms. The other 12 studies were split on the issue, and seven favored the for-profit form with five for the not-for-profit form. Pauly (1987) best summarizes these results when he observed that holding size, quality, and teaching status constant, little difference in the provision of hospital care is attributable to ownership status. The one exception is the operating performance of public not-for-profit hospitals. Zelder (1999) also reviewed 15 studies comparing public and private hospital performance and found compelling evidence that private hospitals are more efficient than public hospitals.

ALTERNATIVE MODELS OF HOSPITAL BEHAVIOR

Accepted alternatives to the profit-maximizing model share a common approach: utility maximization. In practice, profit maximization is just a special case of utility maximization. The only practical difference between the two models is the way in which residual earnings are distributed. Because utility is unobservable, the challenge is to specify a model with an objective function that is observable.

Utility-Maximizing Models

Here, decision makers in a not-for-profit hospital maximize utility subject to a break-even constraint. The objective of the decision makers may be their own utility. In this case, they will operate the hospital to maximize their own pecuniary and nonpecuniary benefits. Nonpecuniary benefits include the prestige and authority that go along with the position. Empirical research has explored many possible elements in the utility function for hospital administrators. The most popular include output and quality, or some combination of the two (Henderson, 2002).

The utility-maximizing approach assumes that the hospital decision maker's objective is to be in charge of the largest or the highest quality hospital possible given the resources available. Studies by Newhouse (1970), Sloan (1980), and Danzon (1982) use this approach to model the behavior of not-for-profit hospital managers. Quality is typically measured by the level of technology, the type of facility and services, the quality of the staff, and the number of specialists. Running a hospital that ranks high in these quality measures provides a great deal of prestige to the manager. Recruiting staff is easier, as is generating charitable donations for further enhancements to quality.

In practice, the assumption of quality maximization is merely a variant of profit maximization (and cost minimization) to support other objectives. Short run profit maximizing behavior may be pursued in order to invest profit in quality. Adding quality in most cases serves to increase costs and shift demand. Quality enhancements are not free and consumers have a demand for quality. Overinvesting in quality improvements begins to produce a higher-quality product that consumers are willing to buy. These models explain certain behavior, such as investment in technology to increase prestige, but they shed little light on the important role that physicians play in the hospital setting (Henderson, 2002).

Physician-Control Models

If physicians are the relevant decision makers, they have a stake in what combination of inputs is used. Staff physicians may have a financial stake in maintaining an efficient operation. In contrast, private practice physicians with hospital admitting privileges may be more concerned about their own productivity than hospital efficiency. Excess hospital capacity enables physicians to maximize their own incomes. Because the prices of other inputs are effectively zero to nonstaff physicians, they have little concern over the productivity or actual prices of the inputs. Thus, any increase in demand is met by increases in hospital capacity rather than increases in physician staff. The excess capacity enables physicians to maximize their use of their own time (Henderson, 2002).

Physician control leads to technical efficiency in production, where the physician faces a zero price for other inputs, and too many other inputs are used relative to physician inputs. This imbalance suggests that physicians are interested in the hospital investing in additional services to increase hospital capacity, such as: interns and residents who provide services for which the physician can charge, additional operating rooms and obstetric facilities, and any other investment that will serve to economize on their own time (Henderson, 2002).

The physician wants the hospital to price complementary services in order to increase demand for physician services. They also want the hospital to provide outpatient services and preventive care. The former reduces the risk of treating nonpaying patients. The latter is time intensive for the physician and is to be avoided.

Certain services provided by physicians and hospitals are somewhat substitutable for one another. As the physician population increases, more services will be provided in the physicians' offices than in the hospital. If payments for health care are based on total price, lower hospital charges mean greater residuals for the physician.

Payment for hospital services is separated from payment for physician services, making the physician neither financially responsible to the hospital nor accountable to the patient for the cost of the hospital portion of care. Any attempt to control costs without the cooperation of physicians has little chance of success (Henderson, 2002).

THE TREND TOWARD MULTIHOSPITAL SYSTEMS

One of the most important trends in the hospital market during the past two decades has been the increase in multihospital systems (Ermann and Gabel, 1984; Morrisey and Alexander, 1987). In 1975, one out of every four hospitals in the United States was part of a multihospital system, which means that the hospitals participated with at least one other hospital that were owned, managed, or leased by a single entity. Merger activity increased dramatically in the late 1980s. More than 1300 separate hospital acquisitions took place between 1989 and 1993 (Danzon, 1994). By 1993, one out of every two hospitals was part of a multihospital system. Today, more than 450 multihospital systems cover 90 percent of all hospitals in the country (Official National Hospital Blue Book, 2000). Except for

Columbia/HCA, a nationwide chain of more than 340 hospitals, most consolidations in the industry have been among hospitals at the local level (Dranove et al., 1995).

The Theory of Consolidation

Mergers, acquisitions, and other forms of consolidation occur in the hospital industry for the same reasons that they occur in any other industry. Horizontal integration allows businesses to: take advantage of economies of scale, reduce administrative costs, and improve customer access to information. Horizontal integration occurs when two or more firms that make the same product combine (Henderson, 2002).

Firms are said to experience economies of scale when the long run average costs fall as the size of the operation expands. If economies of scale are to result in improved efficiency, a number of technical advantages must be realized because of increased size. These advantages may include the ability to secure discounts through bulk purchasing and to take advantage of specialization and division of labor, especially in the use of highly-skilled personnel. Because the case mix differs so dramatically from hospital to hospital, the relationship between cost and output is difficult to measure. Larger hospitals tend to treat more seriously ill patients, and thus have higher average costs (Cowing et al., 1983; Vitaliano, 1987).

The Empirical Evidence on Consolidation

Most of the empirical research on the growth of hospital systems and efficiency is based on data from a time period when cost-plus reimbursements were the standard practice. Under these conditions, hospitals have little incentive to lower costs (Renn et al., 1985; Santerre and Bennett, 1992).

As hospital reimbursement shifted from retrospective to prospective payment beginning in the mid 1980s, the efficiencies of the multihospital system have become more evident. Research by Dranove, Shanley, and Simon (1992) suggests that substantial unexploited opportunities for economies of scale may exist in the hospital industry, especially in smaller markets. Although antitrust policy has shown a tendency to reject efficiency arguments, these potential economies may serve as a justification for future hospital merger activity.

Dranove and Shanley (1995) focus on the marketing strategy used by hospital claims to promote brand name identity. This strategy, similar to the one used by international franchises in the fast food industry, has as its goal to create a perception of standardized quality in the minds of potential customers. Danzon (1994) argues that chains have a comparative advantage in providing information on product quality that customers value in their decision-making process. Given the uncertainties of the hospital market, customers seek out inexpensive information on quality and service. Identification with an established chain of respected hospitals improves customer access to information, in turn increasing demand and allowing higher margins over costs.

Mobley (1997) examines the differences in merger activity between for-profit and not-for-profit hospitals. Her findings indicate that for-profits and not-for-profits seem to have different motives for consolidating. For-profits apparently seek out lucrative niche markets sheltered from competition. In contrast, the not-for-profit acquisitions are more focused on markets where managed care penetration is higher. By consolidating in markets with high managed care penetration, they are better positioned to bargain with managed care plans. Also, for-profit hospitals can take advantage of the economies of scale without having to expand any one facility beyond its maximum level of efficiency. By satisfying the demand of managed care plans for a full range of services, non profit hospitals are better able to compete in these market areas.

Consolidation activity presents a challenge to antitrust policy. If consolidation leads to efficiency gains, then patients could benefit from higher quality care at lower prices. With the volume of consolidation activity that has taken place in the past decade, it is surprising how little consensus surrounds the extent of scale economies in this industry (Henderson, 2002).

SUMMARY

Hospital care tends to be the most expensive aspect of healthcare delivery. Dominated by the private not-for-profit hospital, the industry is responsible for more than one-third of all healthcare spending. Of interest for policy purposes has been the recent increase in consolidations and mergers, particularly the high profile not-for-profit to for-profit conversions. The changes that began in the 1980s pushed hospitals to become competitive and profit oriented. This corporate mentality has led to extensive local marketing, leveraging debt, multihospital chains, and administrators earning salaries rivaling corporate executives.

Key Words

- Horizontal integration
- Competition
- Efficiency

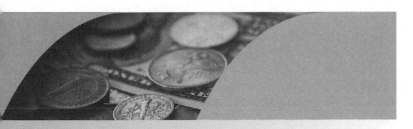

Questions

1. What are the major criticisms related to the for-profit hospital?

2. In theory, describe the different operating characteristics of the for-profit and the not-for-profit hospitals.

3. Does the not-for-profit structure in a hospital eliminate for-profit behavior? Explain.

4. What is a horizontal merger?

REFERENCES

1. AAMC Council of Teaching Hospitals. (1999) *Geographic Listing*. Washington, DC: Association of American Medical Colleges.

2. Alchian, AA and H Densetz. (1972) Production, information costs, and economic organization. *American Economic Review*, 62(5):777–795.

3. Cowing, TG, Holtmann, AG, and S Powers. Hospital cost analysis: a survey and evaluation of recent studies. In Scheffler, RM and LR Rossiter, eds. *Advances in Health Economics and Health Services Research, Vol. 4*. Greenwich, CT: JAI Press; 1983.

4. Danzon, P. (1982) Hospital profits: the effects of reimbursement policies. *Journal of Health Economics*, 1(1):29–52.

5. ——— (1994) Merger mania. *Health Systems Review*, 27(6):18–28.

6. Dranove, D and M Shanley. (1995) Cost reductions or reputation enhancements as motives for mergers: The logic of multihospital systems. *Strategic Management Journal*, 16(1):55–74.

7. ——— and C Simon. (1992) Is hospital competition wasteful? *RAND Journal of Economics*, 23(2):247–262.

8. Ermann D and J Gabel. (1984) Multihospital systems: issues and empirical findings. *Health Affairs*, 3(1):50–64.

9. Feldman, R and B Dowd. (1986) Is there a competitive market for hospital services? *Journal of Health Economics*, 5(3):277–292.

10. Held, P and M Pauly. (1983) Competition and efficiency in the End Stage Renal Disease Program. *Journal of Health Economics*, 2(2):95–118.

11. Henderson, JW. (2002) *Health Economics and Policy*. Cincinnati, OH: South-Western.

12. Johnson-Lans, S. (2004) *A Primer for Health Economics*. Boston: Pearson Addison Wesley.

13. Keeler, EB, Melnick, G, and J Zwanziger. (1999) The changing effects of competition on nonprofit and for-profit hospital pricing behavior. *Journal of Health Economics*, 18(1):69–86.

14. Kessler, DP and MB McClellan. (2000) Is hospital competition socially wasteful? *Quarterly Journal of Economics*, 115(2):577–615.

15. Luft, H et al. (1986) The role of specialized clinical services in competition among hospitals. *Inquiry*, 23(1):83–94.

16. Mayo, J and McFarland, D. (1989) Regulation, market structure and hospital costs. *Southern Economic Journal*: 559–569.

17. Mobley, LR. (1997) Multihospital chain acquisitions and competition in local health care markets. *Review of Industrial Organization*, 12(2):185–202.

18. Morrisey, MA. (1995) *Cost Shifting in Health Care: Separating Evidence from Rhetoric*. Washington, DC: AEI Press.

19. ——— and JA Alexander. (1987) Hospital participation in multihospital systems. In: Scheffler, RM, and LR Rossiter, eds. *Advances in Health Economics and Health Services Research, Vol. 7*. Greenwich, CT: JAI Press.

20. Newhouse J. (1970) Toward a theory of nonprofit institutions: an economic model of a hospital. *American Economic Review*, 60(1):66–74.

21. *Official National Hospital Blue Book* (2000) Atlanta, GA: Billian Publishing Inc./Trans World Publishing, Inc.

22. Pauly, MV. (1987) Nonprofit firms in medical markets. *American Economic Review Proceedings*, 77(2):257–262.

23. ——— and M Redisch. (1973) The not-for-profit hospital as a physicians' cooperative. *American Economic Review*, 63(1):87–99.

24. Renn, SC et al. (1985) The effects of ownership and system affiliation on the economic performance of hospitals. *Inquiry*, 22(3):219–236.

25. Robinson, JC and HS Luft. (1987) Competition and the cost of hospital care 1972–1982. *Journal of the American Medical Association*, 257(23):3241–3245.

26. ——— McPhee, SJ and SS Hunt. (1988) Hospital competition and surgical length of stay. *Journal of the American Medical Association*, 259(5):696–700.

27. Santerre, RE and DC Bennett. (1992) Hospital market structure and cost performance: a case study. *Eastern Economic Journal*, 18(2):209–219.

28. Shalit, SS. (1977) A doctor-hospital cartel theory. *Journal of Business*, 50(1):1–20.

29. Sloan, F. (1980) Internal Organization of hospitals: A descriptive study. *Health Services Research*: 203–230.

30. Sloan, F, Perrin, J, and Valvona, J. (1986) In-hospital mortality of surgical patient: Is there a basis for standard-setting? *Surgery*, 99(4):446–453.

31. Sloan, F. (1988) Defining geographic markets for hospitals and the extent of market concentration. *Law and Contemporary Problems*, 51(2): 165–194

32. Stevens, R. (1989) *In Sickness and in Wealth: American Hospitals in the Twentieth Century.* New York: Basic Books Inc.

33. Vitaliano, DF. (1987) On the estimations of hospital cost functions. *Journal of Health Economics*, 6(4):305–318.

34. Zelder, M. (1999) *How Private Hospital Competition Can Improve Canadian Health Care.* Vancouver, BC: The Fraser Institute.

BIO: UWE E. REINHARDT

Uwe E. Reinhardt was born in war torn Germany and immigrated to Canada where he attended the University of Saskatchewan. After graduation in 1964, he came to the United States to study at Yale University, where he received his PhD in 1970. He also holds an honorary doctorate from the Medical College of Pennsylvania. As an academic, he has taught at Princeton University for his entire career. He is currently the James Madison Professor of Political Economy.

Most of Reinhardt's scholarly work is in health economics. He is on the editorial board of several journals, including *Health Affairs*, *New England Journal of Medicine*, and *Health Management Quarterly*. He is also associate editor of the *Journal of Health Economics*.

Reinhardt's fascination for health economics has led him to become an advocate for the uninsured. Prone to black humor about many health issues, he never jokes about the plight of the uninsured. He firmly believed that health care plays a social role, but is not a constitutional right. It is a right "implied in the social contract… It's not a consumer good. It's a quasi-religious commodity… It's the cement that makes a nation out of people."

Source: Julie Rowner. "MM Interview: Uwe Reinhardt," *Modern Maturity* 37(6) November/December 1994, 64–72.

Health Economics and Policy, 2nd Edition. James W. Henderson. (Cincinnati, OH: South-western, 2002).

CHAPTER 13

The Pharmaceutical Industry

LEARNING OBJECTIVES:

In this chapter, you will learn about:

1. the underpinnings of pharmaceutical drug pricing.
2. how the government intervenes to promote the safety of the population.
3. the health of the market for prescription drugs.

DRUG COSTS

This chapter will help you to understand why drugs are priced as they are and to evaluate the pros and cons of government regulation of the pharmaceutical industry. An understanding of the biopharmaceutical industry requires us to study its market structure, pricing policies, the effects of government regulation, the effects of cost-containment strategies of third party payers, and the role of international competition. The behavior of the industry can only be understood if we are careful to distinguish between short run costs of manufacturing a drug, after it has been developed and introduced into the market, and the long run costs, which include research and development (R&D) costs. In this chapter, we will also consider the effects of new drugs, insurance coverage, and advertising on the demand for prescription drugs.

THE BIOPHARMACEUTICAL INDUSTRY

Biotechnology, which involves research into the nature of fundamental genetic material, is the new facet in the biomedical field. In contrast, products developed by the pharmaceutical industry have historically been based on chemistry rather than biology, and new pharmaceutical products are often called **new chemical entities (NCEs)**. The distinction is becoming blurred

and both industries are now producing therapeutic drugs. Examples of important new biotech drugs are erythropoietin, for the treatment of anemia in AIDS, cancer, and patients undergoing kidney dialysis; and interferons used for treating cancer and multiple sclerosis (Scherer, 2000). In this chapter, we will use the word "pharmaceuticals" to refer to the whole class of biopharmaceutical products.

The Importance of Pharmaceuticals

Even though pharmaceuticals still make up only a small fraction of total healthcare expenditures, the proportion devoted to these products has been increasing rapidly in recent years. Between 1990 and 2000, the proportion of healthcare costs devoted to prescription drugs increased from approximately 5 to 10 percent (Berndt, 2002). Increases in expenditures are partly the result of price increases and partly a result of increases in quantity utilized. The increase in quantity is a

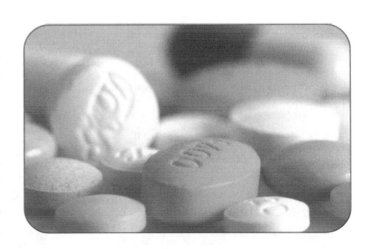

mixture of higher utilization of existing drugs and the purchase of new pharmaceuticals.

MARKET STRUCTURE

Industry Concentration

It is often assumed that firms in the pharmaceutical industry are oligopolies because a few very large companies come to mind when we think of this industry, such as GlaxoSmithKline, Pfizer, Merck, and Johnson & Johnson. However, the biopharmaceutical industry is far less concentrated than is commonly believed and is better described as monopolistically competitive. The firms exhibit behaviors that are typical of this market structure (Scherer, 2000). They engage in vigorous marketing: selling costs are an important component of costs. Ownership of brand names is important, and licensing to foreign distributors is a major source of revenue. Even among the subset of smaller, newer biomedical firms, those which survive over time in the world market tend to gain larger market shares through internal growth or through mergers and acquisitions, although they tend to be located in one country, unlike pharmaceutical giants that are typically multinational corporations.

Competition at the Product Level

Although patent protection confers monopoly power in the production of a drug over the life of a patent, most brand name drugs experience some competition from other drugs used to treat the same illness during their period of patent protection—most new brand name drugs have at least one fairly close substitute at the time of their introduction into the market (Scherer, 2000). It is therefore useful to distinguish between within- and between-patent competition. **Within-patent competition** from imitators occurs after patent expiration and also during on-patent time from firms in countries that do not enforce patent law. **Between-patent competition** from firms developing different products to treat the same diseases may be even more important. One of the implications of the between-patent competition and its effect on the returns from R&D is that it may make changes in patent policy, such as the increase in patent life from 17 to 20 years, less important (Lichtenburg et al., 2002).

Effects of Firm Size on Research & Development Productivity

A number of studies have investigated the effect of pharmaceutical firm size on research productivity. It is widely believed that large firms have advantages in both economies of scale and scope, but there is evidence that the situation is somewhat more complicated (Chandler, 1990). Economies of scope occur when there are positive spillover effects within the firm from having a number of different R&D projects at the same time. A study covering all research projects in ten major pharmaceutical firms over 20 years used data at the level of individual research programs within firms. No evidence of increasing returns to scale or scope per se was found, but complicated sets of interdependencies between economies of scale and scope, and the greater ability of large firms to absorb both intrafirm economies and external spillover effects, appeared to give larger firms an advantage. The net result was that larger firms which conduct more research projects tended to also have more productive research programs (Henderson and Cockburn, 1996). Larger firms were also found to be more likely to undertake research that integrates process and product development.

GOVERNMENT REGULATION OF THE PHARMACEUTICAL INDUSTRY IN THE UNITED STATES

Unlike medical and surgical devices, pharmaceutical products are heavily regulated by the U.S. government, particularly with respect to the extensive testing required by the Food and Drug Administration (FDA) before new products can be launched. A drug receives approval only if it meets the requirements with respect to both safety and efficacy. Another type of regulation is the legal requirement that certain drugs can be purchased only if prescribed by a licensed practitioner. An important question is how much regulation is optimal.

Regulation by the Food and Drug Administration

Federal regulation of the quality of drugs marketed in the United States began with the enactment of the Pure Food and Drug Act in 1906 that created the FDA. The passage of the Kefauver-Harris Act in 1962 greatly strengthened the FDA, which had just gained widespread applause for banning the sedative thalidomide, the source of serious birth defects in Europe. The Kefauver-Harris Act required a more stringent regime of clinical testing to launch both NCEs and generic versions of drugs already on the market. The number of new drugs launched per year declined after 1962 (Johnson-Lans, 2006).

An unintended consequence of the more stringent regulatory climate appears to have been a differential impact on small firms. Smaller firms suffered a decline in both their research productivity and market share. Why this occurred is not clear, but it appears that firms need both breadth and depth of research capacity to be successful in launching drugs when there is a more arduous testing process required for drug approval. Research and Development costs per project have also been shown to decline with firm size (Dimasi et al., 1995).

There is evidence that the largest U.S. pharmaceutical firms actually benefited from the harsher regulatory climate. Declines in their own research productivity were more than offset by the gains in sales resulting from less competition (Thomas, 1990).

In 1971, the government added a proof of efficacy to the requirements for the introduction of new drugs. Overall requirements became more stringent, and by the 1990s the average time from first application to the FDA approval of a drug had risen to over nine years. The following schedule shows the average time required for the development of an NCE in the late 1980s:

1. Discovery of an NCE
2. Preclinical animal testing
3. File application for authorization for human testing (approximate time for discovery, preclinical and application approval: 3.5 years)
4. Phase I clinical testing: test the effects on a limited number of healthy volunteers—test absorption rate, metabolic effects, etc. (average time: 15 months)
5. Phase II clinical testing: administer drug to larger sample of humans—those with conditions the NCE is intended to treat (average time: 2 years)
6. Long-term animal studies (usually concurrent with human testing)
7. Phase III clinical testing: large scale testing to determine efficacy and side effects (average time: 3 years)
8. New drug approval process (average time: 2.5 years) (Dimasi et al., 2003)

Liberalization of the FDA Process

Generic Drugs

When patents expire on brand name drugs, chemically equivalent copies of the drug can be produced. These copies are known as generic versions of the drug or generic drugs. In 1984, the Waxman-Hatch Act was passed, which allowed generic drugs to be introduced with much less burdensome testing requirements. Manufacturers had only to show that the active ingredients in the generic version were the same as those in the patented drug and the drug would be absorbed into the bloodstream within a +/− range of 20 percent. Between 1984 and 1998, the generic share of the drug market increased dramatically from about 19 to 44 percent, in part because of this legislative change (PhRMA, 1998).

Orphan Drugs

The Orphan Drug Act was passed in 1983 and defined **orphan drugs** as those used to treat rare diseases (i.e., those with fewer than 200,000 cases). The purpose of this legislation was to en-courage the production of drugs for which there was little market potential. Firms are given tax breaks, funding help, and exclusive rights to market orphan drugs for seven years, even when they are not on patent. As of May 2003, the FDA had approved orphan status for 240 drugs. However, in many cases the so-called orphan drugs are also used to treat multiple diseases, some of which are far from rare (Johnson-Lans, 2006). From 1998 to 2003, orphan drug prices rose by 40 percent per year compared with an increase of 15 percent per year in nonorphan drug prices. In 2003, the Centers for Medicare and Medicaid Services (CMS) reduced rates of reimbursement to hospitals and doctors for most orphan drugs. In order to keep costs down, Medicare now classifies multiuse orphan drugs like all other drugs and reimburses accordingly. As a result of this change, only four therapeutic drugs are currently reimbursed by Medicare on the basis of their orphan drug status. One of these is Cerezyme, Genzyme's drug for Gaucher's disease. Only about 3500 people take the drug, but in spite of this small population of consumers, it generated $619 million in revenue for Genzyme in 2002 (Elias, 2003).

Compassionate Use of Experimental Drugs

Criticism of the FDA's conservativism led to the adoption of a new drug approval procedure in the 1980s, whereby experimental drugs awaiting approval may be made available to physicians for limited use in treatments for patients in advanced stages of disease. This approval procedure releases drugs for use in the treatment of patients with such diseases as advanced AIDS and late-stage cancer (Johnson-Lans, 2006).

The Prescription Drug User Fee Act of 1992

The Prescription Drug User Fee Act of 1992 caused some acceleration of the approval process by granting the FDA authority to collect fees from firms when applications are filed and when they are accepted. The fees increased the FDA's operating budget, allowing it to act more rapidly. The average time from start of clinical testing to market approval has declined from 98.9 to 90.3 months. This is largely because the approval phase has been shortened from, on average, 30.3 to 18.2 months (Dimasi et al., 2003).

Requirement for Prescriptions (Rx)

A second type of regulation intended to promote the safety of the general public is the requirement that a wide range of drugs be available to consumers only when prescribed by a licensed physician. This regulation is also controversial. One study has found no statistically significant different outcomes in such indicators as rates of poisoning in comparing the United States with other industrialized nations that do not require prescriptions for most nonnarcotic drugs (Peltzman, 1987). Because lower doses of prescription drugs are often available over the counter and anyone can take multiple pills, this does not seem to be a very failsafe method of preventing toxicity.

The argument that the requirement of prescriptions from physicians is not in the public interest is made more plausible when one observes the many near-equivalents to newer prescription drugs that are available without prescription in the over-the-counter (OTC) market (Johnson-Lans, 2006). An unintended negative consequence of the prescription requirement is that consumers may choose higher-cost Rx drugs rather than OTC drugs when their health insurance covers the former. This may result in inflated drug expenditures and extra costs for physician visits.

Liberalization of the Rx Requirement

Beginning in the 1970s, the FDA began to allow the conversion from prescription (Rx) status to OTC status for a limited number of drugs when pharmaceutical companies could prove that even misuse of the drug would not have harmful effects. It is in the insurance companies' best interest to promote OTC status for drugs because the OTC drugs are not usually covered by insurance. The popular allergy medication, Claritin, became available OTC in the United States at the instigation of an insurer, Wellpath, and against the will of both the manufacturer, Schering-Plough, and physician groups (Peterson, 2002). However, pharmaceutical companies may also benefit from their drugs being changed to OTC status. The Waxman-Hatch Act enables companies that have been granted OTC status for a drug to apply for a 3-year exclusive period during which time no other company may market a similar OTC version of the drug. A second advantage to manufacturers of OTC status drugs is that the FDA regulates OTC versions of drugs much less heavily than drugs requiring a prescription (Johnson-Lans, 2006).

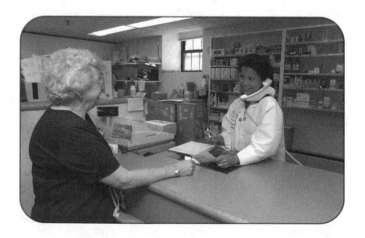

Effects of Regulation on Pharmaceutical Firms' Success

A positive effect of stricter regulation of pharmaceutical products has been found. Firms with home countries imposing higher safety standards in the introduction of new drugs into the domestic market have been shown to benefit in their command over market share in foreign markets (Thomas, 1996). Moreover, stringent regulations with respect to efficacy also seem to positively affect success in world markets. In countries where approval of drugs has an efficacy requirement, firms seem to direct more research toward developing products embodying significant improvements over existing drugs (Thomas, 1996).

DEMAND FOR PHARMACEUTICALS

The demand for pharmaceuticals is affected by the introduction of significant new products, by the substitution of pharmaceuticals for other more invasive treatments, by the aging population, by the expansion of insurance coverage for prescription drugs, and to some extent by the shares of direct marketing to consumers in 1997 (Johnson-Lans, 2006).

Effect of Increased Insurance Coverage for Prescription Drugs

Between 1965 and 1998, the proportion of U.S. prescription drug expenditure that was paid out-of-pocket by consumers decreased from 92 to 26.6 percent. In 1965, private insurance covered only about 3.5 percent of the expenditures on prescription drugs, as opposed to 52.7 percent in 1998 (Department of Health and Human Services, 2000). In addition, there was no Medicaid drug coverage in 1965. With the introduction of the Medicare prescription drug benefit, the share of out-of-pocket payment for prescription drugs will decline even more (Johnson-Lans, 2006).

Third party payment now routinely reimburses a higher proportion of generic drug costs as opposed to brand name drugs in an attempt to make consumers and physicians more cost-conscious. Medicaid also reimburses only the price of the generic drug when substitutes for brand name drugs are available. In this way, insurance companies can affect the balance of generic and brand name drugs utilized by altering relative prices to consumers (Johnson-Lans, 2006).

Effect of Direct Marketing to Consumers

Since 1997, direct marketing of drugs to consumers has been legal in the United States. This makes it possible for drug companies to create a consumer demand for products that physicians might not otherwise recommend. Pharmaceutical companies are particularly likely to aggressively advertise drugs being introduced as substitutes for drugs that are going off patent. Direct marketing to consumers also provides a greater incentive to develop lifestyle products, such as treatment for hair loss or sexual dysfunction. This kind of advertising serves to both provide information and induce demand (Johnson-Lans, 2006).

PRICING ISSUES

No aspect of the medical economy receives more attention today than the prices of prescription drugs, even though the substitution of pharmaceuticals for other medical treatments often involves significant savings to patients in both time and money (Scherer, 2000). Many countries now control the prices of drugs and there are a variety of complicated ways in which this is done (Sherer, 2000). Public policy regarding the pricing of pharmaceuticals for its citizens is more complicated in a country that is also the home of a major pharmaceutical industry, as in the case of the United States—the one that still leads the world in the introduction of new drugs. It is much easier for a country such as Canada, which does not have a major domestic pharmaceutical industry, to regulate the price of prescription drugs. The United States has generally not imposed price controls on pharmaceuticals except for in the 1970s under the presidency of Richard M. Nixon (Johnson-Lans, 2006).

Price Differentials Between Brand Names and Generic Drugs

Once drugs are off patent, generic versions that are chemically identical can be marketed. It is widely believed that generic drugs are sold for lower prices than equivalent brand name drugs, even when produced by the same company. A peculiar phenomenon does exist—brand name drugs are frequently sold at higher prices after the introduction of generic substitutes than before. The reason for this is the decline in price elasticity of demand for the brand name drug after it is off patent. When the generic drug is introduced, the demand for the brand name drug decreases. However, the segment of the market that is loyal to the brand name drug has a demand that is less price-elastic than the total demand for the product during the time it was on patent. The producers of the brand name drug often decide not to compete with the generic version of the drug, but rather to raise brand name prices in response to the decline in demand elasticity (Frank and Salkever, 1992). This strategy seems to be employed whether or not they sell the generic version of the drug in addition to the brand name.

Discounting of Drugs to Third Party Payers

Discounts to insurers below the retail price is another form of price discrimination and one that has become increasingly

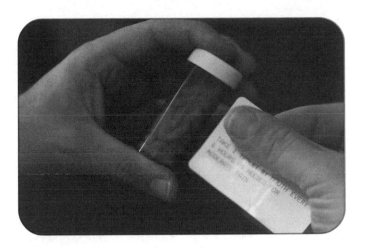

important in the United States in the age of managed care. HMOs and other large insurance companies are able to use their buying power to negotiate price discounts with manufacturers and wholesalers in return for higher rates of insurance coverage for the product or for including the product on an approved list called a formulary list. When Medicare purchases drugs for hospitalized patients, it also negotiates a discounted price with manufacturers. Note that this does not apply to Medicare Part D reimbursement for outpatient drug purchases. Medicaid only reimburses at the generic rate when substitutes are available for brand name drugs. The Department of Veterans Affairs (VA) and the Department of Defense are known for negotiating the lowest drug prices in the United States (Frank, 2001).

Pharmacy Benefit Management Firms

Insurance companies also employ other firms to negotiate for them. **Pharmacy Benefit Management firms (PBMs)** have emerged as service institutions for large insurance companies. PBMs act as intermediaries in the retail market for prescription drugs for insured patients. They both negotiate prices with pharmacists and manage the paperwork. In addition, they make their own formulary lists and obtain discounts from drug manufacturers in return for having their products included on the lists. PBMs also exert pressure on physicians to prescribe lower priced drugs. This has resulted in widespread substitution among brand name drugs. The United States is known for its high priced drugs, but it is not widely known that although its brand name prices are usually the highest in the world, its generic drug prices are among the lowest (Danzon, 1997). Pressure from insurance companies is one of the reasons for the wider differential in price between brand name and generic versions of a drug in this country than in many other parts of the world (Johnson-Lans, 2006).

Price Differences among Countries

The prices of pharmaceutical products vary widely among countries. This phenomenon is not just the result of firms' decisions to engage in price discrimination based on differences in elasticity of demand. It also reflects differences in cost of production. Some countries bear more of the product development. Moreover, governments engage in a wide variety of techniques for controlling drug prices, including direct price controls. A number of governments in countries that have extensive social programs relate their rates of reimbursement for newer patented drugs to prices of the same drug in other nations. Two resulting factors of this are multinational companies charging higher prices in some countries than they otherwise would and withholding marketing new drugs in certain countries, such as India, which has both low income and regulation limiting prices (Scherer, 2000).

Effect of a Country's Pricing Policy on the Launching of New Drugs

Price regulation in domestic markets also affects both the timing and the number of drugs launched in a country (Danzon et al., 2003). Countries that regulate launch prices tend to have the lowest rate of launching new drugs. As part of the process of new drug approval, most countries now have a requirement that third party payers will reimburse for this drug, if introduced. Germany, the United Kingdom, and the United States are exceptions in not having this requirement (Johnson-Lans, 2006).

Effects of Parallel Importing on Price Differentials among Countries

International price differentials tend to be undercut by commercial reimportation of pharmaceutical products manufactured abroad. A review of economics of price discrimination reminds us that price discrimination can only be effective when resale can be prevented among markets. The difficulty in practicing price discrimination based on geographical market segmentation is likely to increase in the future with more trade agreements leading to legal reimporting of drugs manufactured in foreign countries. The commercial reimporting of drugs, called parallel importing, is now permitted within the European Union. Price differentials between drugs sold in Canada and the United States could be reduced somewhat if commercial reimportation of drugs from Canada, currently being challenged, becomes legal (Pecorino, 2002). However, one main source of the current difference in Canadian and U.S. drug prices is the much greater tort liability risk that drug manufacturers face in the United States. It is unclear how this would apply to drugs manufactured in Canada, but sold in the United States (Manning, 1997).

PROFITABILITY OF THE U.S. PHARMACEUTICAL INDUSTRY

Profits are often thought to be higher in the pharmaceutical industry than in most other industries in the United States. This was particularly true during the economic boom of the 1990s. A frequently used measure of profits is the ratio of current earnings to the value of the company's capital stock. This is called the return on equity. The average return on equity in 1998 for the five largest pharmaceutical companies was 42.4 percent, whereas the return on equity for Microsoft in the same year was only 27 percent. The only other company in the top ten largest U.S. corporations with comparable profit levels was Coca-Cola with a return of 42 percent (Folland et al., 2001).

However, because the proportion of cost devoted to R&D and the rate of technological change are substantially higher in the pharmaceutical industry than in most other industries, the return on equity tends to exaggerate the profitability of pharmaceutical firms, given the way R&D expenditures are treated on corporate balance sheets. Measuring current return on equity largely ignores costs already incurred in previous time periods (sunk costs). Scherer maintains that a better measure of profitability is quasi-rents, which are the revenues in excess of the sum of current production costs and the amounts used to defray R&D costs that have already been incurred. This makes sense when we think of the wide disparity between marginal costs of producing another batch of pills and the R&D costs associated with developing and introducing a new drug. Using this approach, Scherer has found profit margins in the pharmaceutical industry to not be significantly higher than the average for other industries (Scherer, 2000).

It is important to take into account the high probability of research ending in products that never reach the market. The failure rate has to be factored in when considering the cost of introducing new chemical entities. Even in the case of drugs that receive FDA approval, only a small proportion provide enough revenue through sales to cover the R&D costs incurred in their development. Of the 100 new drugs introduced into the domestic market in the United States in the 1970s, the top ten products produced 55 percent of the quasi-rents from sales both at home and abroad. These drugs are called blockbuster drugs. Only the top 20 most profitable drugs fully covered their producer's R&D (Grabowski and Vernon, 1990, 1994).

SUMMARY

At the end of the twentieth century, the United States still led the world in the development of new pharmaceuticals, although the costs of developing new drugs had risen dramatically at the same time that managed care imposed downward pressure on the domestic prices of new drugs.

The flow of new products continues to stimulate demand for pharmaceuticals, as does the increase in third party prescription drug coverage. Growth in revenues of U.S. pharmaceutical companies since 1994 has resulted primarily from the increase in volume of sales (Berndt, 2002). Berndt predicts that the ongoing rate of R&D should lead to a continuing flow of new products throughout the next decade.

Key Words

- New chemical entities
- Within-patent competition
- Between-patent competition
- Orphan drugs
- Pharmacy benefit management firms (PBMs)

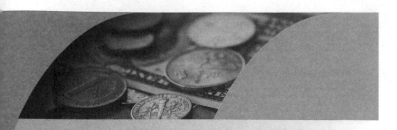

Questions

1. Why might a drug company raise the price of its brand name drug when it comes off patent?

2. Discuss the pros and cons of the conservative stance of the FDA with respect to the introduction of new pharmaceutical products onto the market.

3. Why may a pharmaceutical firm prefer to have its product changed from Rx to OTC status?

4. What factors have contributed to the increase in the cost of successfully launching a NCE?

REFERENCES

1. Berndt, ER. (2002) Pharmaceuticals in US health care: determinants of quantity and price. *Journal of Economic Perspectives*, 16:45–66.

2. Chandler, A. (1990) *Scale and Scope.* Cambridge, MA: MIT Press.

3. Danzon, PM. (1997) Price discrimination for pharmaceuticals: welfare effects in the US and the EU. *International Journal of the Economics of Business*, 4:301–321.

4. Danzon, PM, Wang, TR, and L Wang. (2003) *The Impact of Price Regulation on the Launch and Delay of New Drugs: Evidence from Twenty-five Major Markets in the 1990s.* NBER Working Paper No. 9874. Cambridge, MA: National Bureau of Economic Research.

5. Department of Health and Human Services. (2000) *Report to the President: Prescription Drug Coverage, Spending, Utilization and Prices.* Washington DC: DHHS.

6. Dimasi, JA et al. (1995) R&D costs, innovative output and firm size in the pharmaceutical industry. *International Journal of Economics and Business*, 2:201–209.

7. ——— (2003) The price innovation: new estimates of drug development costs. *Journal of Health Economics*, 22:151–185.

8. Elias, P. (2003) Orphan drugs save lives, but come at a hefty price. *The Seattle Times*, May 26, 2003, p C3.

9. Folland, S, Goodman, C, and M Stano. (2001) *The Economics of Health and Health Care*, 3d ed. Upper Saddle River, NJ: Prentice Hall.

10. Frank, RG. (2001) Prescription drug prices: why do some pay more than others? *Health Affairs*, 20:115–128.

11. Frank, RG and DS Salkever. (1992) Pricing, patent loss, and the market for pharmaceuticals. *Southern Economic Journal*, 59:165–179.

12. Grabowski, HG and JM Vernon. (1990) A new look at the returns and risks of pharmaceutical R&D. *Management Science*, 36:804–821.

13. ——— (1994) Returns on new drug introductions in the 1980s. *Journal of Health Economics*, 13:383–406.

14. ——— and JA Dimasi. (Supplement 2003) Returns on research and development for the 1990s new drug introductions. *PharmacoEconomics*, 20:27–28.

15. Henderson, R and I Cockburn. (1996) Scale, scope and spillovers: the determinants of research productivity in the pharmaceutical industry. *RAND Journal of Economics*, 27:32–59.

16. Johnson-Lans, S. (2006) *A Health Economics Primer.* Boston: Pearson Addison Wesley.

17. Lichtenburg, F. (2002) The effects of Medicare on health care utilization and outcomes. Forum for Health Economics and Policy, *Berkeley Electronic Press*, 5(1):1028.

18. Manning, RL. (1997) Product liability and prescription drug prices in Canada and the US. *Journal of Law and Economics*, 49:203–243.

19. Pecorino, P. (2002) Should the US allow prescription drug reimports from Canada? *Journal of Health Economics*, 21:699–708.

20. Peltzman, S. (1987) The health effects of mandatory prescriptions. *Journal of Law and Economics*, 30:207–238.

21. Peterson, M. (2002) Claritin to sell over the counter. *The New York Times*, November 28, 2002, p. C1.

22. *PhRMA Industry Profile 1998.* Washington, DC: Pharmaceutical Research and Manufacturers of America.

23. Scherer, FM. The pharmaceutical industry. In: Cuyler and Newhouse, eds. *Handbook of Health Economics*, Vol 1B, Amsterdam: Elsevier; 2000.

24. Thomas, LG. Industrial policy and international competitiveness in the pharmaceutical industry. In: Helms, RB, ed. *Competitive Strategies in the Pharmaceutical Industry.* Washington, DC: AEI Press; 1996.

25. ——— (1990) Regulation and firm size: FDA impacts on innovation. *RAND Journal of Economics*, 21:497–517.

BIO: VICTOR R. FUCHS

Victor R. Fuchs' contributions to the field have been so important that many consider him to be one of the founding fathers of health economics. He received his BS in Business Administration from New York University and was awarded his PhD from Columbia University in 1955. After being denied tenure at Columbia University, he worked at the National Bureau of Economic Research (NBER) and the Ford Foundation. After six years at NBER, he joined the faculty at the City University of New York (CUNY) and then Stanford University in 1974. He is currently the Henry J. Kaiser Jr. Professor of Economics at Stanford.

Fuchs saw a research vacuum in the application of the economic perspective to issues relating to health and medical care. Equipped with a boundless curiosity, he garnered the reputation as one of the foremost empirical economists of our time.

One of his most important contributions to the study of health economics came in a 1967 paper published while he was still at the NBER. In that paper, he concluded that a person's health status may be more depended on lifestyle considerations than the level of medical care received. The theme that individual actions matter quickly became part of the thinking of epidemiologists and other health researchers.

Fuchs' research in the early 1970s challenged the commonly held belief that the American Medical Association was responsible for keeping medical care prices artificially high. Several studies testing the economic theory of physician-induced demand led him to conclude that more physicians would actually lead to higher levels of utilization and higher prices. As a tribute to his research contribution, Harvard University Press anthologized 17 of his papers in 1986 under the title *The Health Economy*.

Since Fuchs' move to Stanford, virtually all of his writing has been for general audiences or others with little or no training in economics. His work has been well received by noneconomists because of the straightforward empirical nature to the questions facing our daily lives, such as family, work, education, religion, and health. Calling himself a "radical moderate," he strongly advocates a balanced approach to problem solving. His research may be characterized as positive rather than normative, and he is more comfortable using data to explain factual observations than advancing specific policy measures.

Source: Joseph P. Newhouse, "Distinguished Fellow: In Honor of Victor Fuchs." *Journal of Economic Perspectives* 6(3), Summer 1992, 179–189.

Health Economics and Policy, 2nd Edition. James W. Henderson. (Cincinnati, OH: South-western, 2002).

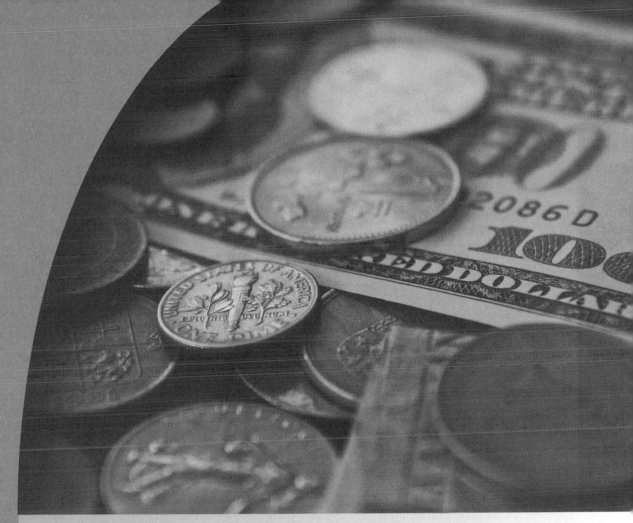

PART VI

EVALUATING THE HEALTHCARE SYSTEM

CHAPTER 14

Economic Evaluations

LEARNING OBJECTIVES:

In this chapter you will learn:

1. the role of economic evaluations in health care.
2. the types of economic evaluations and their uses.
3. the components of a complete economic evaluation.

METHODS OF ANALYSIS

Economic evaluations involve the quantification of changes in health resource utilization due to the introduction of new courses of action. Policy makers are increasingly turning to such analyses to acquire information before making decisions about alternatives in health care (Stoddart, 1982). Such analyses are used by insurers to determine which services to pay for, and government policy analysts use technology assessments to shed light on the economics of new interventions and courses of action (Tengs et al., 1995). Economic evaluations are used to make systematic decisions concerning the allocation of resources in the market. They provide insights into how resources ought to be allocated. In this chapter, we include an overview of the methodology; an introduction to the main components and issues surrounding cost minimization analysis, cost-effectiveness analysis, **cost-utility analysis** and cost-benefit analysis; and guidelines for the use of economic evaluations.

WHAT DO ECONOMIC EVALUATIONS ADDRESS?*

Economic evaluations answer the following questions in order to provide an objective set of criteria for making choices among alternatives given scarce resources:

1. Are health services, etc., worth doing given limited resources? For example, a health department may ask, "Should everyone get a flu shot each year, given that shortages of vaccine can exist?," or clinicians may ask, "Should the blood pressure be checked for every adult who walks into their offices, given the time constraints of the standard office visit?"
2. Are we satisfied with the way health resources are utilized in the different courses of action chosen? For example, a hospital administrator may ask, "Should each and every new diagnostic instrument really be a good purchase?" or an insurer may ask, "Should people request that they receive annual check-ups?"

What Is the Purpose of an Economic Evaluation?

The purpose of an economic evaluation is to compare alternative courses of action that are solutions to the same problem. Without systematic analysis, it is difficult to clearly identify the alternative uses for resources and the opportunity cost of employing one alternative over another in solving a problem. For example, a health department may need to evaluate the

---

*There is a growing literature on economic evaluation in health care. Studies have been conducted by economists, medical researchers, clinicians, and multidisciplinary teams based on one or more of these types of expertise. Although the studies vary in quality, several good introductions to health economic evaluations already exist (Drummond et al., 1997; Gold et al., 1996; Jacobs and Rapoport, 2002; Stoddart, 1982). All of these give a reader a basic interpretation of the nature of economic evaluation and an appreciation of the decision making required at all levels. This chapter is a supplement to such sources and the reader is encouraged to explore these other materials as needed.

efficiency of a diabetes prevention program and a bicycle helmet initiative in reducing the number of disability days in a population (Messonnier et al., 1999). It can also determine if the course of action is worthwhile (i.e., whether to address problem or not)—and whether changes are worth the cost (Scheffler and Paringer, 1980).

Economic evaluations provide an objective way to determine resource allocations from an individual, community, or societal viewpoint. There are two general viewpoints to an economic evaluation: private and societal. The private perspective is focused on the individual, an organization, or a set of organizations. A healthcare organization may be interested in the cost benefit of a palliative care program versus traditional medical protocols. In this case, the firm is not interested in the transfer payments that may result by participation because these are not paying for resources being utilized. Instead, the firm is concerned with its own direct and indirect costs of the courses of action and their associated outputs (see Table 14-1). The societal view includes all persons so that the opportunity cost of the various courses of action can be taken into account. In terms of a palliative care intervention, this would include all direct and indirect costs of the courses of action and the transfer payments that may be involved as well, because they reflect the opportunity costs of pursuing one course of action versus another for the population as a whole (Drummond et al., 1997).

Economic evaluations link the alternative courses of actions' inputs and outputs and provide a comparative analysis of alternative courses of action in terms of the value of their inputs and outputs. Without such an analysis, it is difficult to objectively justify the value for the money invested in an alternative. The real cost of any alternative isn't measured by the budgetary allocations, but by the health output achieved through some other alternative which has been foregone by committing resources or inputs to the alternative in question. This cost is the opportunity cost of the alternatives considered and is compared to the alternative's benefits. Figure 14-1 depicts a diagram of the process (Drummond et al., 1997).

TYPES OF ECONOMIC ANALYSES

The identification and measurement of costs is similar across the economic evaluation methods and are discussed later in the chapter. However, the type of output from the alternative courses of action can vary significantly across the methodologies. Four types of evaluation methods illustrate this concept. A summary of the various types are seen in Table 14-2.

Cost-Minimization Analysis

In this case, outputs of the courses of action are identical (or at least assumed to be so), and costs only are considered. For example, a comparison of the common output of interest is the number of successful procedures at a day surgery center versus

TABLE 14-1 Types of Outputs of a Course of Action.

Outputs: changes in physical, social, or emotional role function

Health: changes in natural units (e.g., reduction in disability days, reduction in blood glucose levels) — **Utility:** changes in the quality of life of patients and their families (e.g., QALY or Healthy Years) — **Benefits:** changes in resources utilized

Direct — 1. Organizing and operating services within the health sector for original or unrelated conditions; 2. Related activities of patients and their families (e.g., savings in expenditures or leisure time input)

Indirect — 1. Savings in patients' or families' lost work time

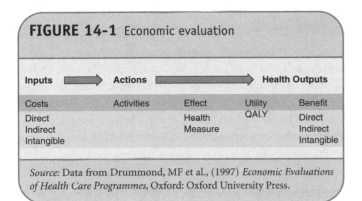

FIGURE 14-1 Economic evaluation

Source: Data from Drummond, MF et al., (1997) *Economic Evaluations of Health Care Programmes*, Oxford: Oxford University Press.

performing the procedures at an outpatient center of a hospital (Evans and Robinson, 1980). In this example, we may find an identical number of procedures performed, but possibly different costs. The principle decision rule is focused on the costs per procedure successfully performed, where the least cost course of action is determined to be the efficient choice (Drummond et al., 1997).

Cost-Effectiveness Analysis

In this case, the output of the courses of action is common across alternatives, but the alternatives have varying degrees of success in achieving the output. An example would be the comparison of different diabetes prevention programs (Gray, 2000; Elixhauser, 1989). The decision rule is based on the cost per unit of output or output per unit of costs. The decision maker selects the course of action that yields the most output

per dollar spent or the least cost per output. The latter decision is used when the decision maker is working within a given budget. This implies that there is a single, common affect that is constrained, and that the alternatives are within the same range of scale. This analysis can be done considering any courses of action with a common output. The worth of the courses of action is assumed to be positive. Here, we assume that the courses of action have value for the population and are efficacious (Drummond et al., 1997).

The outputs can be health effects directly or measures that show improvements in health status. For instance, one can compare a prevention program versus a chronic care program in terms of disability days saved per dollar invested in each program (Hatzriandreou et al., 1988; Tengs et al., 1995). In cost-effectiveness analysis, there is a dominant dimension of success that is considered. If there is an equivalent level of effectiveness, it is best to perform a cost-minimization analysis. Also, it is important to be open to the possibility of using more sophisticated analyses, such as cost-benefit analysis, if there is more that one dimension of effectiveness.

In conducting a cost-effectiveness analysis, several data issues should be addressed. First, the analyst must assure that there is a random allocation of patients to groups. Second, if the investigation is looking at existing literature, it is important to see how studies relate to provider expertise and the patient caseload in question. Third, a sensitivity analysis, discussed later in the chapter, can eliminate the need for clinical trials (especially in extreme effectiveness issues). However, if a clinical trial is used, the investigator must assure that the analysis of the

TABLE 14-2 Summary of Economic Evaluation Methods.

Method	Measure of costs of courses of action	Identification of outputs	Measurement of outputs
Cost-minimization analysis	Dollars	Identical across alternatives	None
Cost-effectiveness analysis	Dollars	Single, common output among alternatives, achieved in varying degrees	Natural units, e.g., disability days reduced or reduction in blood glucose levels
Cost-utility analysis	Dollars	Single or multiple outputs, not necessarily common across alternatives, and achieved in varying degrees	Healthy days or QALYs
Cost-benefit analysis	Dollars	Single or multiple outputs, not necessarily common across alternatives, and achieved in varying degrees	Dollars

clinical trial doesn't cause any deviation of normal working practices (Drummond et al., 1997). Fourth, it is more meaningful if the results of the cost-effectiveness analysis are compared to some standard for the problem being investigated (Laupacis, 1992; Doubilet, 1996).

Cost-Utility Analysis

This is often considered a special case of cost-effectiveness analysis, where the output of the courses of action is valued commonly across alternatives, but the alternatives have varying degrees of success in achieving the value of the improvement in the output. In this case, both the output and the worth of the courses of action are measured. An example of such an analysis is the improvement in the **quality-adjusted life years (QALYs)** due to a diabetes intervention versus usual care. This technique is preferred by many economists because it incorporates the utility of the output (Torrance and Feeney, 1989), or in other words, the preferences of the patients or the population considered (Drummond et al., 1997).

Utility, introduced in Chapter 2, is the value or worth of a specific health state and can be measured by the preferences of persons for any set of health states. Utility of the health output is different than the health output itself. It brings in quality of life adjustments for treatment output, while providing a common denominator for comparing the costs and outputs of different alternatives. The measure for utility is seen in the measures of healthy days or QALYs. Here, the length of time of the health state is adjusted though a utility scale 0–1, with 0 being the worst value of the health state) (Sintonen, 1981; Williams, 1981). The decision rule is to choose the alternative with the lowest cost per healthy year equivalent (HYE) or QALY.

Willingness to pay for an additional QALY can be determined from community-based surveys (O'Brien and Viramontes, 1994; Hirth et al., 2000) However, these surveys need to follow procedures similar to those for contingent valuation studies discussed later in the chapter (Gold et al., 1996).

Cost-Benefit Analysis

In this case, the output of the courses of action may not be a single common effect, but may be multiple effects which may or may not be common to the alternatives. For example, one could compare a health promotion programs for youths with a chronic care intervention for the elderly on a variety of output dimensions. We could perform a cost-effectiveness analysis on multiple effects to determine a decision rule where an alternative is superior on all or a majority of dimensions in the comparison (Drummond et al., 1997).

Alternatively, we could develop a method to combine multiple effects into one common valuation. Here, the measure of value is the dollar, translating effects into the dollar value benefit of life years gained, improved productivity, more convenience, etc. This comparison of dollar costs or dollar benefits is cost-benefit analysis. This results in a ratio of dollar costs to dollar benefits or the sum of net social benefits, where net social benefits equals social benefits minus social costs. The decision rule is to choose the course of action that has the greatest net social benefits (Drummond, 1981). Benefits will be large enough so that those who gain could theoretically compensate the losers and everyone is made better off (i.e., the Pareto principle) The preferred method is to maximize net benefits rather than the B/C ratio because the ratio can be misleading depending on how benefits and costs are categorized. In this method, the absolute benefit is determined, which is the value of the resources used compared to the value of the resources saved or created. The implicit assumption is that the courses of action are compared to a do-nothing alternative. However, in health care, because there are usually costs involved in do-nothing states, this comparison is not usually done in practice. The valuation of the benefits can be done through the human capital method or the contingent valuation framework. The instrument used depends on the purpose of the evaluation (Drummond et al., 1997).

The human capital method places a value on the opportunity cost of lost time, such as lost wages or the value of replacement workers for duties without a wage (Viscusi, 1978). For example, if a person is in the labor force and needs to take time off from work due to disability, then the value of the loss of work would be measured using the wage rate. If the person is out of the labor force and has a disability that reduces the level of productivity, then the value of the loss is the replacement worker to complete the tasks no longer completed by the person in question. In many ways, this approach is debatable among economists because wages underestimate the total loss of time, particularly leisure time. Also, the approach favors the employed rather than those out of the labor market, which leads to inequities in compensation (Drummond et al., 1997).

Contingent valuation is what a person would hypothetically pay if they could achieve the benefits from specific interventions. In other words, it is the willingness to pay for improved care (Shogren et al., 1994; Donaldson, 1999). Because this is a hypothetical approach, the surveys obtaining the value of the preferences must be clearly defined with the following characteristics:

1. They must clearly state the characteristics of the alternative.
2. They must identify other goods and services that are competing for the person's household budget.
3. They must explain that spending would be reduced on other goods or services if more is spent on the alternative in question.

4. They must explain that the cost of the alternative would be seen with an increased tax or price.

5. There must be a follow-up survey to obtain the rationale for respondents' valuations of the alternatives. (Drummond et al., 1997)

Because the Pareto principle is satisfied hypothetically, cost-benefit analysis traditionally doesn't account for income redistribution. Redistribution takes the form of taxes and transfers and can be criticized as inefficient. In practice, such as in welfare reform plans, redistributional effects have been explicit, where the most general procedure is to classify the benefits and costs on a person-by-person or group-by-group basis. The redistribution depends on the relative weights applied to benefit distribution, and redstributional criteria may override efficiency criteria because projects are usually constrained so that the poor cannot be made worse off (Drummond et al., 1997).

Cost

Cost is the value of the resource used for any particular course of action. The type and scope of costs depend on the analysis viewpoint (e.g., society, government, patient, employer, and program agency). When in doubt, it is best to go to the broadest or societal viewpoint. In any viewpoint, the costs include the direct and indirect costs of the course of action considered. Direct costs are the actual expenses incurred by participating in the alternative. This includes the medical expenses, transportation costs, and other training costs that can be part of the alternative. Indirect costs are the productivity losses associated with the course of action, which reflect the opportunity costs of using one alternative and forgoing another (Luce and Elixhauser, 1990; Olsen, 1994; Jacobs and Fassbender, 1998). For example, this could include the waiting time for appointments, and transportation time as part of the participation in a course of action. In the private perspective, transfer costs are also included because they reflect changes in payments for in-

dividuals, providers, or organizations. From the societal view, direct and indirect costs are included, but transfer costs are not because these are not resources used. A summary of cost types is seen in Table 14-3.

If the magnitude is small, then the study can merely identify it. Overall, economic costs go beyond simply listing expenditures, because opportunity costs need to be reflected, such as the need to consider other nonmarketed resources (e.g., leisure time, donated space, etc.). Costs can be estimated in a variety of ways. For example, values are imputed for nonmarket items. Leisure time may be measured by earnings lost by the corresponding wage rate (Drummond et al., 1997).

Discounting

Discounting accounts for the differential timing of costs and outputs of particular courses of action under consideration over multiple periods of time. People place a higher value on benefits in the present period than in future periods. The discount rate reflects this social rate of time preference and expresses this preference for the present over the future periods. Therefore, all costs are discounted to their present value (Drummond et al., 1997). The discount rate is equal to the social rate of time preference, which denotes that people prefer their benefits now rather than in the future. Empirically, this rate is equal to the interest rate on a risk-free asset, such as government treasury bills. Discounting nonmonetary benefits has been controversial, especially for prevention or health education programs (Viscusi, 1995). Specifically, the approach diminishes the impact of health promotion programs that have a longer time horizon until outputs are recognized to their fullest, but favors those programs that have more immediate impacts.

Sensitivity Analysis

Overtime, the sensitivity analysis technique has become virtually mandatory in economic evaluations, and improvements in

---

TABLE 14-3 Summary of Types of Costs Considered in an Economic Evaluation.

Direct costs	1. Organizing and operating costs related to the course of action. (e.g., capital costs, supplies, labor, equipment, utilities) 2. Costs borne by the patients and their families (e.g., out-of-pocket expenses, patient and family input into course of action, psychological costs)
Indirect costs	Time lost from work due to participation in course of action or due to illness related to course of action
External/societal costs	Costs borne externally to the health sector, patients, and their families

the technique have emerged with more statistically-inclined economists working on the method. Sensitivity analysis is a means to determine the robustness of the evaluation recommendations under circumstances where the estimates are controversial or uncertain (Briggs et al., 1994; Briggs and Sculpher, 1995). It clearly identifies uncertain or controversial estimates in a study, and a presents an exposition of the ways in which different assumptions about how the estimates impact the study results. In terms of when to use this analysis, consider estimates that are subject to debate due to:

1. new variables being used (e.g., value of life scales)
2. variations in data collection or measurement (e.g., per diem costs)
3. controversy in value judgments (e.g., choice of discount rate)

(Drummond et al., 1997)

The basic approach is to set upper, expected, and lower ranges of evaluation estimates based on varying the parameters in question. These estimates can be obtained from:

1. empirical evidence from other research
2. current practice in the literature
3. judgments from decision makers in the study

(Drummond et al., 1997)

The course of action that is dominant under most or all of the scenarios would be the one chosen. This analysis also allows the analyst and audience to understand which conditions would make the course of action inefficient relative to other alternatives. It may be necessary to specify a threshold set of study result estimates that are above or below which a course of action may no longer be efficient.

ASSESSMENT OF AN ECONOMIC EVALUATION

A sound economic evaluation has the components seen in a good empirical research study. These are outlined in Table 14-4. While these questions are not raised to create hypercritical users of economic evaluations, they do provide a means to quickly identify the strengths and weaknesses of the economic evaluation. It is highly unlikely that every economic evaluation would include all of the components noted below. Even with study weaknesses, the reader may find that the method of the evaluation considered compares well with alternative approaches to the same problem (Drummond et al., 1997).

A more thorough explanation of the questions from Drummond et al. (1997) is below:

1. **Was a well-defined and operational question formed?**

    In answering this question, the reader would determine if there is a comparison of alternatives, a descrip-

> **TABLE 14-4** Critical Questions When Reviewing an Economic Evaluation.
>
> 1. Was a well-defined and operational question formed?
> 2. Was a complete description of the alternative courses of action provided?
> 3. Was there evidence of program effectiveness?
> 4. Were all important costs and outputs for each course of action identified?
> 5. Were costs and outputs measured accurately?
> 6. Were costs and outputs valued credibly?
> 7. Were costs and outputs adjusted for differential timing?
> 8. Was an incremental analysis of costs and outputs performed?
> 9. Was a sensitivity analysis performed?
> 10. Did the presentation of the findings include all issues of concern to the users of the analysis?
>
> *Source:* Data from O'Brien B. (1995) Principles of economic evaluation for health care programs. *J Rheumatol*, 22:1399–1402; and Drummond, MF et al., (1997) *Economic Evaluations of Health Care Programmes*. Oxford: Oxford University Press.

tion of the viewpoint of the analysis, and whether both costs and outputs of the alternatives are considered.

2. **Was a complete description of the alternative courses of action provided?**

    In answering this question, the study should address the "whom?", "what?", "where?", and "at what frequency?" questions, and whether a do-nothing alternative was considered.

3. **Was there evidence of program effectiveness?**

    In answering this question, the reader must determine how effectiveness is established. For example, was the effectiveness derived from current literature, and how strong is this determination from the literature?

4. **Were all important costs and outputs for each course of action identified?**

    In answering this question, the program description and viewpoint of the analysis should provide enough evidence that the appropriate costs and outputs are included. For example, a study may be considered where a reduction in the highway speed limit reduces traffic-related deaths and injuries, but also includes a higher wage for the transportation workers. It is also important that the outcomes of interest be identified clearly for the reader to judge the appropriateness of the economic evaluation method being used. The reader needs to know whether the outputs are health effects (appropriate for cost-effectiveness analysis), changes in the quality of life of the participants (appropriate for cost-utility analysis), or what the overall value is of the outcome created (appropriate for cost-benefit analysis).

5. **Were costs and outputs measured accurately?**

   For example, the measurement of operating costs of a particular course of action may include such things as 500 examinations, 100 hours of physician time, 200 hours of nursing time, rental for 1000 square feet of clinic space, etc. Costs borne by the participants may be measured by medicines purchased, time lost from work or leisure, and travel time to the treatment location.

6. **Were costs and outputs valued credibly?**

   It should be remembered that costs are a valuation of the resources depleted by a particular course of action. Costs are usually valued in local currency based on a prevailing process of resources and can be taken from operating budgets. All current and future program costs are measured in constant dollars of some base year in order to put the values in real terms.

7. **Were costs and outputs adjusted for differential timing?**

   Different courses of action may have different time profiles of costs and outputs, but the comparison of the alternatives must be made at one point in time and the timing among programs must be taken into account. For example, the main benefits of an influenza vaccine program are immediate, while the benefits of a colorectal screening program are not identified until well into the future. In order to compare the different timing of the courses of action considered, the reader should determine if discounting is used as described in section 14.2.

8. **Was an incremental analysis of costs and outputs performed?**

   For a more meaningful comparison across courses of action, the reader should be able to determine the additional costs that one course of action imposes over another, compared to the additional outputs (e.g., health effects, utilities, or benefits) it yields. In practice, the impact of most courses of action add to both costs and outputs, especially compared to when no course of action is taken.

9. **Was a sensitivity analysis performed?**

   Every evaluation will have some degree of uncertainty or methodological controversy. For example, "What if a discount rate of 6 percent were used rather than 3 percent?" Or "What if the rate for childhood vaccinations is 10 percent lower than considered in the analysis?" Evaluators will often rework the analysis by employing different assumptions or estimates in order to test the sensitivity of the conclusions of the analysis to such changes. This technique is discussed in section 14.2. If large variations in the assumptions or parameters yield little variations in the results of the study, then the reader would have more confidence in the original results.

10. **Did the presentation of the findings include all issues of concern to the users of the analysis?**

    A good study should begin to help the user interpret the results in the context of their own particular situation. For example, many users of these analyses are interested in the bottom line, such as whether or not to purchase a new MRI system. The analysis can be presented in such a way that it is explicit about the viewpoint being considered and that it identifies how particular costs and benefits may vary by location. For example, the purchase of a new MRI system may vary by whether the system would be a replacement unit in an existing imaging center or one that will be part of a newly-converted center.

SUMMARY

This chapter attempted to provider the reader with an introduction to the nature of economic evaluation and the main types of economic evaluations, as well as the elements of a sound economic evaluation. The complexity of the analysis must match the breadth of the questions posed in determining the type of economic evaluation techniques. Cost-minimization analysis and cost-effectiveness analysis assume that the courses of action considered are worth considering, while cost-benefit analysis and cost-utility analysis actually determine the worthwhileness of the alternative through mechanisms for preference revelation. Different approaches can be used together for complicated problems and at times a cost-benefit analysis is performed of the economic evaluation itself, because these analyses are costly to perform.

Key Words

- Willingness to pay
- Cost-utility analysis
- Quality-Adjusted Life Year (QALY)

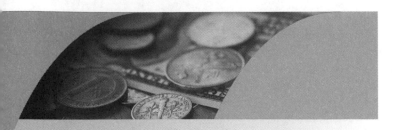

Questions

1. You are asked to compare the outputs and costs of two cardiac interventions that affect the severity of the illness and the patient's survival rate. What evaluation method would you use and why?

2. You are asked to evaluate three medical interventions that reduce the number of deaths due to congestive heart failure. Among these interventions, there are no influences on the patient's quality of life. What evaluation method would you use and why?

3. You are asked whether a new drug to combat congestive heart failure symptoms should be used. What evaluation method would you use and why?

4. How would you account for the differential timing and costs between a health promotion intervention and a treatment regime? What are the pros and cons of using this technique?

5. In practice, the social rate of time preference is measured as the interest rate on a risk-free asset. Do you think that this interest rate is appropriate? Why or why not?

REFERENCES

1. Briggs, AH et al. (1994) Uncertainty in the economic evaluation of health care technology: the role of sensitivity analysis. *Health Economics*, 3:95–104.

2. Briggs, AH and MJ Sculpher. (1995) Sensitivity analysis in economic evaluation: a review of published studies. *Health Economics*, 4(5):355–371.

3. Donaldson, C. (1999) Valuing benefits of publicly-provided health care: Does "ability to pay" preclude "willingness to pay"? *Soc Sci in Med*, 49:551–563.

4. Doubilet, P. (1996) Use and misuse of the term "cost-effective" in medicine. *New England Journal of Medicine*, 314:253–256.

5. Drummond, MF. (1981) Welfare economics and cost-benefit analysis in health care. *Scottish Journal of Political Economy*, 28:125–145.

6. Drummond, MF et al. (1997) *Economic Evaluations of Health Care Programmes*. Oxford: Oxford University Press.

7. Elixhauser, A. (1989) The cost effectiveness of preventive care for diabetes mellitus. *Diabetes Spectrum*, 2:349–353.

8. Evans, RG and GC Robinson. (1980) Surgical day care: measurements of the economic payoff. *Canadian Medical Association Journal*, 123:873–880.

9. Gold, MR, Siegel, JE, Russell, LB, and MC Weinstein (eds). (1996) *Cost-Effectiveness in Health and Medicine*. New York: Oxford University Press.

10. Gray, A et al. (2000) Cost effectiveness of an intensive blood glucose control policy in patients with type 2 diabetes: economic analysis alongside randomized controlled trial (UKPDS 41). *British Med J*, 320:1373–1378.

11. Hatzriandreou, EI et al. (1988) A cost effectiveness analysis of exercise as health promotion. *AJPH*, 78:1417–1421.

12. Hirth, RA et al. (2000) Willingness to pay for a QALY: in search of a standard. *Medical Decision Making*, 20:332–342.

13. Jacobs, P and K Fassbender. (1998) The measurement of indirect costs in the health economics evaluation literature. *Int J Tech Assess in Health Care*, 14:799–808.

14. Jacobs, P and J Rapoport. (2002) *The Economics of Health and Medical Care*, 5th Edition. Sudbury, MA: Jones and Bartlett Publishers.

15. Laupacis, A et al. (1992) How attractive does a new technology have to be to warrant adoption and utilization? Tentative guidelines for using clinical and economic evaluations. *Canadian Medical Association Journal*, 146:473–481.

16. Luce, BR and A. Elixhauser. (1990) Estimating costs in economic evaluations of medical technologies. *Int. J. of Tech Assess in Health Care*, 6:57–75.

17. Messonnier, ML et al. (1999) An ounce of prevention...What are the returns? *Am J Prev Med*, 16:248–268.

18. O'Brien, B. (1995) Principles of economic evaluation for health care programs. *The Journal of Rheumatology*, 22:1399–1402.

19. O'Brien, B and JL Viramontes. (1996) Willingness to pay: a valid and reliable measure of health state preference? *Medical Decision Making*, 14:289–297.

20. Olsen, JA. (1994). Productivity gains: should they count in health care evaluations? *Scottish Journal of Political Economy*, 41(1):69–84.

21. Scheffler, RM and L Paringer. (1980) A review of the economic evaluation of prevention. *Med Care*, 18:473–484.

22. Shogren, JF et al. (1994) Resolving differences in willingness to pay and willingness to accept. *AER*, 84:255–270.

23. Sintonen, H. (1981) An approach to measuring and valuing health states. *Soc Sci in Med*, 15c:55–65.

24. Stoddart, GL. (1982) Economic evaluation methods and health policy. *Evaluation and the Health Professions*, 5(4):393–414.

25. Tengs, TO et al. (1995) Five-hundred life-saving interventions and their cost-effectiveness. *Risk Analysis*, 15:369–390.

26. Torrance, GW and D Feeny. (1989) Utilities and quality-adjusted life years. *Int J Tech Assess in Health Care*, 5:559–575.

27. Viscusi, WK. (1978) Labor market valuations of life and limb. *Public Policy*, 26:359–85.

28. _____ Discounting health effects for medical decisions. In: Sloan, F, ed. *Valuing health care: costs, benefits and effectiveness of pharmaceuticals and medical technologies*. New York: Cambridge University Press; 1995:123–145.

29. Williams, AH. Welfare economics and health status measurement. In: van der Gaag, J and M Perlman, eds *Health, Economics and Health Economics*. Amsterdam: North-Holland; 1981:271–281.

BIO: JOSEPH P. NEWHOUSE

After receiving his PhD from Harvard in 1969, Joseph P. Newhouse spent the next 20 years of his professional career at RAND Corporation. As senior staff economist and head of its economic department, he designed and directed the RAND Health Insurance Experiment, arguably the most important social experiment in health insurance policy in the United States.

While at RAND, Newhouse also served on the faculties of the RAND Graduate School and the University of California at Los Angeles School of Medicine. Returning to Harvard in 1988, he is currently the John D. MacArthur Professor of Health Policy and Management and serves as the director of the Division of Health Policy Research and Education. In addition to his appointment in the Faculty of Arts and Sciences, he is a member of the faculties of Harvard's Medical School and School of Public Health, and the Kennedy School of Government. Under his direction in 1992, Harvard created an interdisciplinary PhD program in health policy encompassing these four areas of study.

Newhouse's curriculum vita lists almost 250 publications, including articles in the top journals in the fields of economics, statistics, and medicine. He has been listed in all three editions of *Who's Who in Economics* as being among the most cited economists from 1970 to 1992. He is the founding editor of the *Journal of Health Economics* and serves as a member of the editorial board, associate editor, and referee for numerous others, including the *American Economic Review*, *Journal of Economic Perspectives*, and the *New England Journal of Medicine*.

As principle investigator in a number of research projects, he has generated more than $100 million in grants and contracts from the Department of Health and Human Services, Health Care Financing Administration, and the Agency for Health Research and Quality, to name a few. Newhouse was recognized for the distinguished contribution to the field of public policy and management with the David N. Kershaw Award and the Prize of the Association for Public Policy and Management in 1983.

Newhouse has become a central figure in health policy research and education in the United States. His current research focuses on several natural experiments with the incentive structure of the federal Medicaid program and project for the Bureau of Labor Statistics to improve the consumer price index for medical care.

Source: Harvard faulty book Web site and Joseph P. Newhouse Curriculum Vita.

Health Economics and Policy, 2nd Edition. James W. Henderson. (Cincinnati, OH: South-western, 2002).

Comparing Healthcare Systems

ELEMENTS OF A HEALTHCARE SYSTEM

A healthcare system consists of organizational units and processes by which a society determines the choices concerning the production, consumption, and distribution of healthcare services (Johnson-Lans, 2004). The structure of a healthcare system is important because it answers basic questions, such as what to produce and who should receive the services produced. At one extreme, the systems may be totally centralized by the government and the government makes these choices; in another extreme, the choices can be made by the market through the interaction of consumers and producers of healthcare services.

From a societal point of view, it is difficult to determine whether a centralized or decentralized health system is superior. A normative statement of that kind entails the value judgments and tradeoffs that are involved. A centralized authority with complete control may be more capable of distributing services more uniformly and have a greater ability to exploit economics of scale and scope. At the same time, it may lack the competitive incentive to innovate or respond to varied consumer-voter demands; also, a centralized authority may face high costs of collecting information about consumer needs (Johnson-Lans, 2004).

Alternatively, a healthcare system that is decentralized, such as the market place or a system of local governments, may provide more alternatives and innovations, but results in diseconomies of scale and scope and lack of coordination. Determining the best structure for a healthcare system involves quantifying the value society places on a number of alternatives and sometimes competing outcomes, such as choice, innovation, uniformity, and production efficiency. Indeed, alternative systems throughout the world exist because people place different values on each of the various outcomes (Reinhardt, 1996). Reflecting the tradeoffs involved, most health systems today are neither purely centralized nor decentralized, but are mixed economies. It is important to keep in mind the decision-making processes in the various countries to understand how the healthcare systems work.

Healthcare systems are huge, complex, and constantly changing as they respond to economic, technological, social, and historical factors. For example, the healthcare system in the United States involves: over 800,000 physicians and dentists, about 2 million nurses, approximately 7000 hospitals, over 80,000 nursing homes and mental retardation facilities, thousands of health insurers and government agencies, and millions of people involved in the production and consumption of health care (Johnson-Lans, 2004). Because of the complexity of healthcare systems, many people have a difficult time understanding how the systems function.

Types of Systems

No two healthcare systems are identical, although many share characteristics that allow us to develop typologies which are useful in analysis of any particular system. It must be noted that while typologies are useful in that they allow us to simplify complex reality and focus on the most important aspects, they must always be viewed as a heuristic tool, not a full representation of reality. The specific configuration of any health system depends on a multitude of factors, such as politics, culture, demographics, historical events, and social structures inherent to a specific country. Societal goals and priorities develop over time and shape all social institutions and values, which themselves are fluid and changeable (Johnson-Lans, 2004).

Despite widespread variation among the healthcare systems of developed nations, at the root they represent variants or combinations of a limited number of types. Typologies here can be useful in simplifying a variety of cross-cutting dimensions, but one must be cautious in interpreting them because they represent ideal types of institutional characteristics. Real world healthcare systems are considerably more complex.

For initial comparative purposes, several typologies used to classify healthcare systems are introduced here. The first classification scheme centers on the dimension of the degree of government involvement in funding and provision of health care. At one extreme is the potential of a completely free-market system with no governmental intervention, while at the other extreme is a tax-supported governmental monopoly of provision and funding of all healthcare services. Although in reality neither extreme exists, along the continuum are three models that together represent the core types of healthcare systems operating in developed countries (Johnson-Lans, 2004).

As illustrated in Figure 15-1, the private insurance or consumer sovereignty model is that with the least state involvement in the direct funding or provision of healthcare services. This type is characterized by the purchase of private health insurance financed by employers and or individual contributions that are task oriented. The basic assumption of this approach is that funding and provision of care is best left to market forces. These types are most clearly represented by the

United States and until recently by Australia, but many systems contain some elements of this type.

The second basic type of health system is the social insurance (or Bismarck) model. Although there is significant variation as to organization, this type is based on a concept of social solidarity and characterized by a universal insurance coverage generally within the framework of social security. As a rule, this compulsory health insurance is funded by a combination of employer and individual contributions through nonprofit insurance funds, often regulated and subsidized by the state. The provision of services tends to be private, often on a fee-for-service basis, although there may be some public ownership of factors of production and delivery. Germany, Japan, and the Netherlands are viewed as examples of this type of system. Singapore, with its compulsory MediSave program, is a variation on the theme of social insurance (Johnson-Lans, 2004).

The third type, and the one which might approach the government monopoly in its pure form, is the National Health Service (NHS or Beveridge) model. This model is characterized by universal coverage funded out of general taxation. Although this model is most identified with the United Kingdom, New Zealand created the first National Health Service in its 1938 Social Security Act which promised all citizens open-ended access to all healthcare services they needed free at the point of use. The provision of health services is solely under the auspices of the state, which either owns or controls the factors of production or delivery. Although they have all moved away from the pure model to varying degrees, the United Kingdom, Sweden, and New Zealand are examples of the NHS model (Johnson-Lans, 2004).

Financing Methods of Various Countries

Because the time and amount of medical treatment costs are uncertain from an individual's consumer's perspective, third party payers, such as private insurance and the government, play a major role in the healthcare economy.

Also, third party payers are responsible for managing the financing risk of purchasing medical services. A third party payer can face a much lower level of risk than does an individual consumer because it can pool its risk among various subscribers by operating on a large scale. The law of large numbers states that while individual events may be random and unpredictable, the average outcome of many similar events across a large population can be predicted fairly accurately. For example, an insurance firm can predict the appendectomy rate by judging from past experiences involving a large number of people, while an individual may not be able to predict the risk of appendicitis. A risk-averse consumer is made better off by making a certain present payment to an insurer for coverage

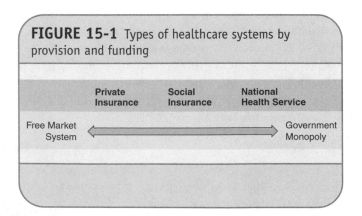

FIGURE 15-1 Types of healthcare systems by provision and funding

	Private Insurance	Social Insurance	National Health Service	
Free Market System	←——————————————————→			Government Monopoly

against an unforeseen medical event, rather than facing the possibility of paying some unknown medical costs (Johnson-Lans, 2004).

Third parties make the healthcare system much more complex because the source of third party financing and the method of reimbursement must be worked into the model. If the third party payer is a private insurance company, the consumer pays a premium in exchange for some amount medical coverage. As part of the health insurance plan, the consumer may be responsible for paying a deductible, a copayment, or coinsurance. The deductible provision requires the consumer to pay the first $X of medical expenses, after which the insurer is responsible for reimbursement. With a coinsurance provision, the consumer pays a fixed percent of the expense at each medical visit. The copayment is the fixed amount of money the consumer pays at each medical visit (Johnson-Lans, 2004).

When a government agency or public insurance company acts as a third party payer, the financing of medical care insurance usually comes from taxes. Premiums and taxes differ in the way risk is treated and in the voluntary nature of the payment (Bodenheimer and Grumbach, 1992). Premiums are voluntary and are paid according to the risk category of the insured. Taxes are mandatory and are paid regardless of risk category.

Some alternative methods of financing can be ascertained by examining the different methods used in Canada, Germany, and the United Kingdom (Raffel, 1997; Blank and Baruau, 2004). These countries are chosen because many features of the United States financing system have been derived from these countries.

Canada

Canada has a compulsory national health insurance (NHI) program administered by each of the ten provinces. Each province has its own unique type of administration. The NHI provides first dollar coverage with no limits on the amount of medical care received during a consumers' lifetime. Each province finances the program through taxes. In addition, the Canadian government provides up to 40 percent of cost sharing and makes hospital construction grants available to the provinces. Private insurance is available for some forms of health services, but not services covered under the NHI. Because the public sector is responsible for the NHI, there are no marketing costs, no allocation of profits, and no determination of who to cover (Johnson-Lans, 2004).

Germany

The Socialized Health Insurance Program (SI) in Germany is based on government-mandated financing by employers and employees. The premiums of unemployed individuals and their dependents are paid by former employers or come from public sources (e.g., public pension funds). **Sickness funds**, which are private nonprofit companies, are responsible for collecting funds and reimbursing healthcare providers and hospitals. Statutory medical benefits are comprehensive and there are small copayments for some services. Affluent and self-employed persons can purchase private health insurance coverage (Johnson-Lans, 2004).

The United Kingdom

Mechanic (1995) and others refer to the healthcare system in the United Kingdom (UK) as a public contracting model because the government contracts with various providers of healthcare services on behalf of the people. The UK healthcare system under the auspices of the National Health Service (NHS), offers universal health insurance coverage financed through taxation. The NHS provides **global budgets** to district health authorities (DHAs). Each district health authority is responsible for assessing and prioritizing the healthcare needs of about 300,000 people and then purchasing the necessary healthcare services for public and private healthcare providers. Hospital services are provided by nongovernmental trusts, which compete with themselves and with private hospitals for DHA contracts. Community-based primary care providers also contract with DHAs. In addition, general practitioner fund holders apply for budgets from the DHAs and with the budgets service a group of at least 5000 patients by providing primary care and purchasing elective surgery outpatient therapy and specialty nursing services. There is some limited competition among the general practitioner fund holders for patients (Johnson-Lans, 2004).

SUMMARY OF VARIOUS HEALTHCARE SYSTEMS

The essential features of the Canadian healthcare system are national insurance, free choice of healthcare provider, private production of medical services, and regulated global budgets and fees for healthcare providers. The dominating features of the German healthcare system include socialized health insurance financed through sickness funds, negotiated payments to healthcare providers, free choice of provider, and private production of healthcare services. In the case of the United Kingdom, the distinguishing characteristics include restrictions on the choice of provider, public contracting of medical services, global budgets for hospitals, fixed salaries for hospital-based physicians, and capitation payments to general practitioners. The pluralistic healthcare system in the United States contains a system of private production, but relies more heavily on a fee-for-service method. In addition, American

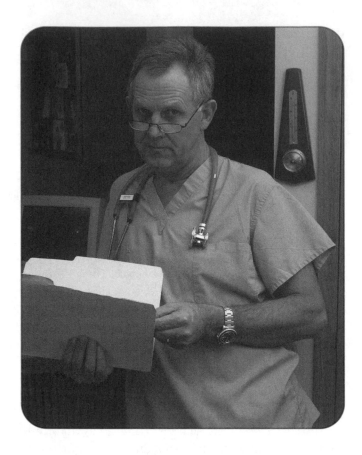

healthcare providers are reimbursed by many types of payers including the government and private insurance firms—in contrast to the **single payer system** of Canada, Germany, and the United Kingdom.

PERFORMANCE OF THE U.S. HEALTHCARE SYSTEM

An aggregate assessment of the U.S. healthcare economy is performed and compared to the performance of a select group of healthcare systems around the world.

Overall Assessment

Prices and expenditures on various medical services continue to rise, but the increase has slowed a bit in recent years. The transition to managed care healthcare delivery has helped to promote some cost savings in various medical care markets, but has also resulted in some rationing of care. Choices of physician, hospital admissions, and selection of pharmaceutical products, while limited under the fee-for-service system, have all been greatly limited by the movement to managed care in the healthcare system. Whether managed care organizations have been able to curb the excesses brought on by unlimited fee-for-service plans of the past or have unnecessarily denied care remains a heated issue and an area for future research. Another issue currently debated is whether or not the cost sav-

ings under managed care can be attributed to the growth of managed care, to a one-time phenomenon, or to the beginning of a long-term trend of slower growth in healthcare expenditures (Johnson-Lans, 2004).

It also seems that competition in the healthcare sector may have created the beginning of its own destruction. For example, cherry picking and red-lining of benefits in the private insurance industry take place because of competition. Quantity-setting behavior in the physician services industry and the medical arms race in the hospital industry are also a result of competition. The debate over the relative merits of competition in the healthcare sector will continue. A position of that debate is taken up in the chapter on healthcare reform (Johnson-Lans, 2004).

Other Healthcare Systems

Now we look at how the United States healthcare system compares to others around the world. It will be interesting and informative to examine how the United States compares to other countries in terms of healthcare expenditures, the utilization of medical care, and healthcare outcomes.

We learned that lifestyle and environmental factors play an important role in determining health status and the demand for medical care. People may try to compensate for risky lifestyle behaviors, such as poor diet or lack of exercise, by consuming healthcare services. This would cause the demand for health care to increase and result in an increase in overall expenditures in health care.

Information on medical utilization shows that perhaps the high medical care spending in the United States results in a relatively large amount of inpatient and physician office visits. An examination of the medical utilization data suggests just the opposite, however. In particular, the United States has only 124.9 hospital admissions per 1000 population in 2000, compared to 226.8 in Germany, and 231.0 in France during that time. Only Japan and Canada had lower rates than the United States. A similar profile is seen for physician visits. Therefore, medical utilization does not explain the high aggregate expenditures in the United States (Johnson-Lans, 2004).

Comparatively high healthcare expenditures with lower utilization rates lead many analysts to believe that medical prices in the United States must be significantly higher than in other countries. Others argue that that the underlying cause may be due to differing quality in health care across countries. Specifically, the quality of medical care may be higher in the United States, thus accounting for the higher prices. Although anecdotal evidence suggests that waiting times are lower in the United States than in other countries, true quality indicators are difficult to derive due to measurement errors.

In summary, nearly 15 percent of the U.S. population is without health insurance coverage throughout the year. In contrast, nearly universal coverage exists in the other countries studied. The government in the United States is responsible for financing about 45 percent of all healthcare spending. The comparable figure for other countries is approximately 90 percent. (Anderson 1997). In the United States, healthcare spending as a fraction of GDP is higher, medical utilization is lower, lifestyle choices are poorer, and infant mortality rates are higher, relative to the other countries considered. Many analysts believe that these findings are a result of the lack of universal coverage in health insurance in the United States; in other countries, the government plays a more dominant role in the delivery of health care. Many analysts also believe that the United States would have similar statistics as other counties if universal coverage and greater government involvement existed in the health economy (Johnson-Lans, 2004).

MEDICAL TECHNOLOGY IN CANADA, GERMANY, THE UNITED KINGDOM, AND THE UNITED STATES

The availability of technology has a profound effect on the healthcare costs and the availability of medical care. Technologies such as drugs, medical devices, and procedures may offer cost savings or higher quality services.

Four stages are associated with the development and diffusion of medical technology. According to the National Science Foundation, the first stage, basic research, is defined as research for the advancement of knowledge without commercial motivations. Basic research produces new medical knowledge about areas in biomedical sciences, for example. In the second stage, applied research, the basic knowledge is applied to yield solutions for the prevention, treatment, or curing of diseases. At the clinical investigation and testing stage, new medical technologies are tested on human subjects—the benefits and safety of the technologies are tested at this point. The final stage, diffusion or imitation, involves the commercial introduction, adoption, and spreading of medical technologies (Johnson-Lans, 2004).

Health policy analysts have expressed concern that the unconstrained healthcare markets result in medical technologies that offer low benefits at high costs (Aaron, 1991). To control costs, many countries have adopted policies to either directly or indirectly control the adoption and diffusion of medical technologies. Public control can be found at any one or all four stages associated with the invention and diffusion of medical technology (Banta and Kemp, 1982). For example, hospital budgets are limited in Canada and Great Britain partly to indirectly control the proliferation of expensive medical

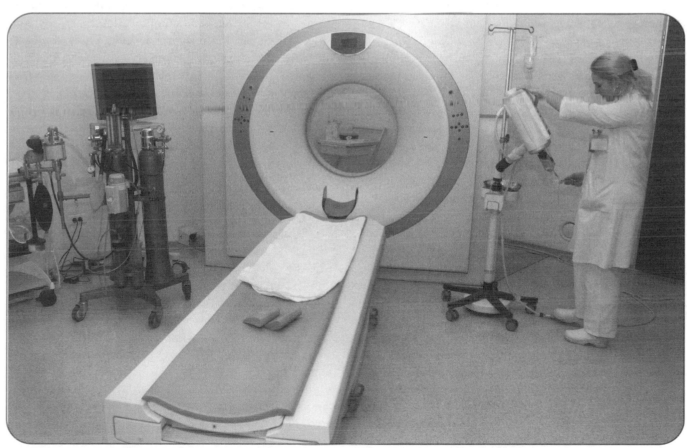

technologies. It is argued that the limited budgets create a financial incentive for hospital administrators to economize on medical technologies offering low benefits at high costs. At the other extreme, the adoption and diffusion of technology are determined more by market forces in the United States. Germany, on the other hand, has taken a middle position between the two extremes with some limited control over the proliferation of new medical technologies (Rublee, 1989).

Reinhardt, Hussey, and Anderson (2002) provide some evidence on the relative availability of different medical technologies in several countries. Several implications can be drawn from their study. First, given the greater reliance on market forces, the data show a greater availability of medical technology in the United States than in the three other countries. For example, the United States has nearly 50 percent more magnetic resonance imagers (MRIs) per million people than the United Kingdom and more than four times more than Canada. In addition, only Germany had more computed tomography (CT) scanners per million people than the United States. There is also a much greater prevalence of coronary artery bypass procedures (CABG), coronary angioplasty procedures, and patients undergoing dialysis in the United States than in the other three counties. Second, the data suggest that to some degree that the relative availability of medical technologies in Germany tends to fall somewhere between the United States and the other two countries. Besides having the most CT scanners, Germany has the second greatest number of MRIs and persons undergoing dialysis and coronary angioplasty. Germany, however, is last among the four countries in terms of coronary bypass procedures. Third, it is difficult to conclude from the available information whether or not medical technologies are overprovided in the United States or underprovided in the other three countries. In fact, a different level of medical technology could be optimal for each country because of differing social values (Rublee, 1994). Cost-benefit analysis, cost-effectiveness studies, or outcomes research would be necessary to draw any definitive conclusions on this issue. Finally, the availability of medical technology in itself indicates little about the overall effectiveness of the healthcare system. To determine overall healthcare system effectiveness, a host of factors must also be considered, including the quantity and quality of other medical inputs.

THE CASE OF SINGAPORE

The pressure to contain rising medical costs has brought considerable attention to Singapore's healthcare system due to its reliance on **medical savings accounts**. Current figures suggest that Singapore spends between 3 to 4 percent of GDP on health care. This is far lower than the 13 percent that the United States spends. Some attribute the ability of Singapore to control healthcare spending to the cost containment incentives that arise with medical savings accounts (Johnson-Lans, 2004).

According to Barr (2001), the Singapore health system is composed of three basic institutional arrangements. The MediSave program is a compulsory savings plan that forms the basis for the individual savings accounts. The contribution rates range from 6 to 8 percent of monthly income and are shared between the employee and employer. Self-employed individuals must pay the entire amount and caps are placed on monthly contributions, which prohibit more affluent individuals from accumulating unreasonably high savings balances. MediSave accounts are used primarily to finance inpatient hospital care and strict payment schedules are in place to protect accounts from being depleted too quickly (Johnson-Lans, 2004).

To protect individuals from the financial burden of a major illness, a catastrophic illness insurance plan, call MediShield, is available. This insurance plan is optional and pays for 80 percent of hospital expenses after a rather substantial deductible has been met, such as $1,000 per year. The third institutional component is the MediFund, which is an endowment established by the government to finance healthcare needs of the poor (Johnson-Lans, 2004).

Barr (2001) contends that the ability of the Singapore healthcare system to contain costs can only partially be explained by the implementation of medical savings accounts. Strict government controls on inputs and prices along with the rationing of medical care have played an even greater role in controlling costs. Other explanations include a relatively young population and the existence of a number of traditional Chinese medical practitioners that are not funded under the government-sponsored healthcare programs, thus the government does not have to pay for their services.

CONSUMER SATISFACTION WITH THE HEALTHCARE SYSTEM IN CANADA, GERMANY, THE UNITED KINGDOM, AND THE UNITED STATES

People in various nations count on their governments to choose and support the healthcare system that best promotes efficiency and equity given their historical background, cultural system, and political beliefs. One question is whether people in these countries are satisfied with their current healthcare system. In an attempt to answer such a question, a number of public opinion polls have tried to estimate the degree of consumer satisfaction with the present healthcare system in a number of nations.

Recently, Blendon and others (2001) cited various opinion polls involving interviews of random samples of households in a variety of countries, including Canada, Germany, the United Kingdom, and the United States. Participants were asked if they were satisfied with the present healthcare system in their respective countries. Several findings from these polls are worth noting.

In terms of overall satisfaction, the German system was superior, but only in a slight margin relative to that of the United Kingdom. Fifty-eight percent of the German households were satisfied with their system compared to 57 percent in the United Kingdom. The German system has a healthcare system characterized by a universal social insurance program. The comparable rates for Canada and the United States are 46 percent and 40 percent, respectively, suggesting that people in the United States are the least satisfied with their current healthcare system. However, if the poll results only consider the poor, the relative ranking changes with the United Kingdom on top with a 67 percent satisfaction rate, and the rate for Germany falling to 52 percent. Among the poor, the United States healthcare system fares a bit better with 47 percent of the poor satisfied relative to 40 percent of the poor in Canada satisfied with their healthcare system.

If the poll results were confined to the elderly, the poll rankings change once again. The United Kingdom healthcare system is superior with 69 percent of the elderly satisfied with their own healthcare system and the United States ranks second with 61 percent of the household satisfied. This could possibly be due to the fact that the elderly in the United States have Medicare, which is a universal health insurance plan for this demographic group. Canada fared the worst, with only 48 percent of older citizens satisfied with their healthcare system.

Public opinion polls may not accurately reflect the success or failure of a healthcare system or provide a complete representation of the quality of life in a nation. For example, low levels of education and income may cause individuals to be generally dissatisfied with their environment. How people feel about the operation of the healthcare system relative to the functioning of the overall economic system might provide a more accurate indicator of public satisfaction. In addition, unbeknownst to the public, the structure of a healthcare system may not account for the poor performance of the medical sec-

tor. The poor performance of a medical care system may be due to inadequate or inefficient allocation of income, resources, or adverse lifestyles. Also, from a general welfare perspective, individuals may be very satisfied with other aspects of the economy, but dissatisfied with aspects of the health economy. These tradeoffs may not be seen in opinion polls solely focusing on the health economy. These aspects should be considered when assessing the overall quality of healthcare systems.

SUMMARY

Every healthcare system must answer two basic questions concerning the allocation of medical resources and the distribution of medical care services. These questions are: what to produce and who should receive the services produced. Some systems rely on centralized decision making, whereas others answer the basic questions through decentralized processes. Healthcare systems are complex largely because third party payers are involved.

Important elements that make up a healthcare system are the financing, reimbursement, and production methods, and the degree of choice over the healthcare provider. Medical care is financed by out-of-pocket payments, premiums, and/or taxes. Medical care providers are reimbursed on a fixed or variable basis. The production of medical care may take place in a for-profit, nonprofit, or a public setting, and medical care providers may operate independently or in large group practices. Choice of provider may be limited. All of these features are important because they influence the operation and performance of the healthcare sector. The United States healthcare system is very pluralistic. For instance, considerable variation exists in the financing, reimbursement, and production of medical care.

Key Words

- Single payer system
- Sickness funds
- Medical savings accounts
- Global budgets

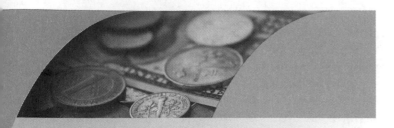

Questions

1. Identify four basic healthcare systems discussed in the chapter.

2. What are the advantages and disadvantages of a single payer system?

3. What are the chief areas of efficiency and inefficiency in the German healthcare system?

REFERENCES

1. Aaron, HJ. (1991) *Serious and Unstable Condition: Financing America's Health Care.* Washington, DC: The Brookings Institution.

2. Anderson, GF. (1997) In search of value: an international comparison of cost, access, and outcomes. *Health Affairs,* 16:163–171.

3. Banta, HD and KB Kemp, eds. (1982) Introduction. In: *The Management of Health Care Technology in Nine Countries.* New York: Springer, 1–9.

4. Barr, MD. (2001) Medical savings accounts in Singapore. *Journal of Health Politics Policy and Law,* 26:709–726.

5. Blank, RH and V Burau. (2004) *Comparative Health Policy.* New York: Palgrave Macmillan.

6. Blendon, RJ, Kim, M, and JM Benson. (2001) The public versus the World Health Organization on health system performance. *Health Affairs,* 210–220.

7. Bodenheimer, T and K Grumbach. (1992) Financing universal health insurance: taxes, premiums and the lessons of social insurance. *Journal of Health Politics, Policy and Law,* 17:439–462.

8. Johnson-Lans, S. (2004) *A Health Economics Primer.* Boston: Pearson Addison Wesley.

9. Mechanic, D. (1995) Americanization of the British NHS. *Health Affairs,* 14:51–67.

10. Raffel, MW, ed. (1997) *Health Care and Reform in Industrialized Countries.* University Park, PA: Pennsylvania State University Press.

11. Reinhardt, UE, Hussey, PS, and GF Anderson. (2002) Cross-national comparisons of health systems using OECD Data, 1999. *Health Affairs,* 21:169–181.

12. ——— (1996) Economics. *Journal of the American Medical Association,* 275:23–25.

13. Rublee, DA. (1989) Medical technology in Canada, Germany and the United States. *Health Affairs,* 8:178–181.

14. ——— (1994) Medical technology in Canada, Germany and the United States: an update. *Health Affairs,* 13:113–117.

BIO: JOHN K. IGLEHART

Mr. Iglehart received his BS in journalism at the University of Wisconsin in 1961. After four years with the Milwaukee Sentinel, he spent six years with the Associated Press in Chicago and was promoted to night city editor. In 1969, he took a position with the *National Journal* in Washington, DC, where he is still one of their contributing editors.

In addition to the numerous articles he has written in health and medical journals, Iglehart is the journalist in residence at the Harvard School of Public Health and national correspondent for the *New England Journal of Medicine.* He also guided the creation of *Health Affairs.* Under his direction, the journals;' circulation has risen above 10,000—the largest for a journal of its type. *Health Affairs* has become a highly respected journal among academicians, policymakers, and journalists. Faculty all over the country are using the journal as a textbook in their health economics classes.

Iglehart is widely known for his research on the medical care delivery systems of Canada, Germany, and Japan.

Source: Project HOPE Website (http://www.projhope.org/HA/aboutha.htm). *Health Economics and Policy,* 2nd Edition. James W. Henderson. (Cincinnati, OH: South-western, 2002).

Healthcare Reform

REFORM INCENTIVES

As we live longer, the incidence of chronic diseases such as heart disease, dementia, and arthritis increase dramatically. We can also expect continued improvement of life-extending technologies, such as mechanical ventilation, artificial resuscitation, and artificial nutrition and hydration. Using these technologies on sicker patients leads to spiraling costs. Quality and access are important, but the overriding issue is costs on the current environment. In this chapter, we explore the nature of reform in the United States, the goals of the reform, and alternative reform strategies.

THE NATURE OF REFORM

The debate over medical care reform is not a new one. Every Congressional session since 1916 has generated at least one piece of federal legislation proposing to modify the system in some way. These issues have remained the same in that quality, access, and affordability are important and needed to be considered, but in recent years the debates have risen to a new level of intensity. In the arena of public opinion, the spiraling costs of health care in the past two decades coupled with the growing number of uninsured and underinsured has created a new level of concern for reform of the system (Henderson, 2002).

Recent polls show that approximately three-fourths of Americans are personally satisfied with the health care that they received, rating it excellent or good (Blendon et al., 1995; Donelan et al., 1999; Robinson, 2000). However, in the same polls, 80 percent of the respondents stated that the system needs some form of reform to make it work better. The respondents are expressing a desire for guaranteed access and lower costs. The policy dilemma is that these two desires are competing and it is not possible to satisfy both completely.

To understand the most recent push for reform, we must understand the forces behind the reform movement (Musgrave, 1993). Some focus on the poor and the elderly as the catalysts for reform, while others note the growing proportion of the uninsured who have restricted access to the private medical care system. These groups are important factors in the reform movement; however, the real incentives for reform are coming from the middle class and businesses.

The middle class perceives itself as being only one paycheck away from bankruptcy and charity care due to limited resources. They are the class that is demanding action because they are the ones that are feeling the pressure. Many middle class members are afraid to change jobs due to the fear of being without insurance coverage during the typical waiting period before employer-based coverage begins for a particular job. Even though insurance plans are required to accept subscribers transferring into plans regardless of insurability, the insured must still pay under the former employer for insurance until the waiting period expires. Most workers are also feeling the rise of insurance premiums through larger payroll deductions. For this group, government involvement means the financial burden will be shifted to wealthy taxpayers or business (Henderson, 2002).

Health insurance benefits are perceived as a big problem for most businesses. With annual premiums rising each year, employee health benefits are often larger than the firms' profit margins. As wages lag behind benefits, workers are becoming increasingly dissatisfied with their disposable income. A strong growing sentiment among businesses is that health benefits should become part of the government's responsibility. Most policy makers would be willing to accept this responsibility in order to control this large and growing sector of the economy (Henderson, 2002).

THE GOALS OF REFORM

The challenge facing decision makers is one of attempting to satisfy unlimited demands placed on the finite resources available to society. Medical care must be placed in the context of other goals considered important by society: national defense, education, environmental protection, just to name a few. To a large extent, these are competing goals. The single-minded pursuit of one goal can lead to ever-increasing expenditures in a given sector. In establishing spending priorities, health and medical care have a significant advantage over other goals. The needs of this sector can be dramatized by citing individual cases where human welfare is involved and consequently spending priorities are easily shifted toward this sector.

Three issues must be addressed when setting out policies to reform the medical care system: who is affected, what is affected, and who pays for the access to the care. It is important to examine reform proposals by these dimensions to see how they satisfy the three criteria (Henderson, 2002).

Who Is Affected?

Most participants in the reform debate agree that the question revolves around universal coverage. Our concern over fairness in the system prompts discussions about the transition from the current system to the new system—whatever it will be.

Expanded access will require, at least initially, additional funding. Policy makers, by now sensitive to voter preferences, are wary of grandiose schemes that require large tax increases in their implementation. Concern over the costs of any change may necessitate the phasing in of access over a number of years, which leads to issues in delayed coverage for deserving groups, such as the poor, disabled, or people of various racial and ethnic classes. Even with these concerns, the policy makers have focused on incremental reforms.

Improved access to care may be accomplished with a mandatory system featuring centralized control of the third party payment system. An example of the **single payer system** would be the Canadian model, which is a universal benefits package and limits the choices available to those who can pay for additional care by making private insurance unable to cover the services that are covered by the governmental program.

Alternatively, expanding coverage to marginal groups defines a different form of universal coverage. For example, private insurance reform could provide small business owners, their employees, and dependents access to group health insurance by purchasing through cooperatives that offer group insurance at affordable rates. The incremental approach presents a dilemma. Relaxing mandated benefits for small businesses leads to a system where individuals have different levels of coverage based on their individual characteristics, such as income or employment opportunities. In other words, reforms geared to enhancing **social welfare** can easily lead to an multi-tiered system of coverage. This is a question for society as to whether or not it would accept these outcomes (Henderson, 2002).

What Is Affected?

The next step is to define a basic benefit package. Reformers who suggest benefit packages that are less generous than those in private health insurance plans are accused of rationing care. This rationing is just an explicit allocation of scarce resources, if viewed economically. In the economic context, the basic benefits package is defined as nothing more than an exercise in establishing priorities, determining how much money is to be spent, and allocating the funds to provide services according to the ranked priorities.

While the decision-making process sounds straightforward, there are competing demands which make the process very difficult. Opinions vary on how the rank ordering of services should be applied—whether one uses medical guidelines or cost-effectiveness analyses as the determining criterion. For example, one group may focus on providing all essential care, while another may decide that only necessary care should be considered (Eddy, 1991; Hadorn, 1991).

Even though we must live with the ethical consequences of such medical system reforms, we also need to finance the system. When part of the system is collectively financed, it may be feasible to envision a benefits plan that is less generous than one in the private market, even though this tiered framework may not satisfy everyone's social ideal. Although such a system is not equitable to all, it is still welfare enhancing because more people have access to a collectively-provided plan (Henderson, 2002).

Who Finances the System?

Most healthcare systems have some form of collective funding though a combination of taxes and insurance premiums. These multiple funding streams imply that it is difficult to build in some natural discipline that is necessary to produce an efficient operation.

Every reform plan must face the concerns of states, affordability, and overall spending. Inevitably, expanding access and providing generous benefits will cause costs to dramatically increase. Individuals spending their own money will react differently from those spending public money in terms of how much they are willing to pay for a reform effort. Normally, the burden of obtaining care falls on the individual, but under certain conditions, it is socially responsible to collectively provide for those who cannot provide for themselves. The issue is really the distribution of the burden of the collectively-provided care. Several questions must be answered before a reform is implemented: Is medical care primarily an individual or collective responsibility, and who bears the cost increase of the reform? (Henderson, 2002).

INDIVIDUAL STATE INITIATIVES

The real battle of reform is fought on the state level. With healthcare costs at the state level rising to over 35 percent of state budgets, the stakes are high for the states. While the federal legislation is being developed at a slow pace, individual states are drafting legislation within their borders to improve their medical care systems and control cost increases. Some significant state initiatives are outlined below (Henderson, 2002).

The Oregon Health Plan

One of the most innovative approaches to healthcare reform attempted to date may be the Medicaid experiment in the state of Oregon. It was controversial because of explicit rationing of services, but had few opponents in the state. Its planners used input from many interest groups, such as patients, providers, payers, and suppliers and held numerous public forums for debates and discussion of various aspects of the plan. After three years of work and one unsuccessful attempt at getting the necessary federal waivers, the state was given the approval to put the plan into effect in 1993. This made Oregon the first state to expand coverage of state-funded benefits to a large number of recipients by limiting the services available.

The original goal of the Oregon Health Plan was to provide health insurance coverage for all state citizens through either a private health insurance plan or Medicaid. To maintain budgetary restraint, the plan set out to ration care by limiting a range of services covered under the basic benefits package. This aspect of the plan is the most controversial. It is a clear case of politics versus economics. The amazing part of the process is that policy makers were able to make choice politically feasible.

The reforms process began with the Oregon Health Services Commission placing over 10,000 diagnoses and treat-

ment into roughly 700 diagnoses/treatment regimes. Using input from over 50 town hall meetings across the state attended by over 1000 citizens, the diagnosis/treatment classes were ranked according to community preferences, effect of treatment on quality of life, and medical effectiveness. After the rank ordering was performed, the list was turned over to the actuaries from Coopers & Lybrand accounting firm to determine the cost of providing care to the citizens of Oregon. Finally, the legislature determined how much money the state could afford to spend on the plan.

The legislature decided to provide a generous package of care equivalent to a typical group plan. Most preventive care—including physical exams, mammograms, PAP smears, and pediatric eye exams and fluoride treatments—was made part of the plan. Also included are dental care, noncosmetic surgical services, hospice care, prescription drugs, and psychiatric services. Specifically, it was determined that the first 585 services would be funded. (Mahar, 1993). The Oregon Legislature faced the reality of the economic tradeoff and remained firm in its commitment. The result is a plan that broadens access to health care at the expense of limited covered services. This sort of pragmatism is unusual given the political pressure on elected officials.

Critics of the approach argue that the process was flawed from the beginning because the diagnosis/treatment rankings were a result of politicians bowing to pressure from disease constituencies and other special interest groups instead of the stated criteria. Others argue that the plan's provisions determine who lives and dies—valuing life in a somewhat arbitrary fashion. Early results were not encouraging. Medicaid spending rose under the new plan compared to early versions. To pay for expanded coverage, the legislature had to levy a 2 percent tax on the gross receipts of healthcare providers, shifting the costs of the plan to private insurance consumers. Attempts at future reform were defeated in 2002 when the electorate voted 4–1 against a state-level single payer plan.

While Oregon made a serious attempt at expanding services to its indigent population, it may not serve as a prototype for the nation due to its relatively homogeneous population. Oregon has approached the problem of administration by systematizing its process. Rather than a haphazard rationing scheme that we have accepted nationally, the state has embraced an open approach. How it performs over time will be important in determining the direction of national reforms.

MinnesotaCare

After years of study and many legislative setbacks, Minnesota legislature passed a comprehensive medical reform law in 1992. MinnesotaCare was a complex piece of legislation providing basic medical benefits for low-income families at subsidized rates and modifying insurance standards to lower the cost to small businesses. Begun as a model plan to provide medical care to pregnant women and small children, MinnesotaCare has evolved into a comprehensible system of stateside healthcare delivery.

In 1987, the Minnesota legislature passed a model healthcare reform bill that provided basic care to pregnant women and young children under the age of eight. Two years after the bill was enacted, the legislature voted to extend the age of eligibility for children to age 18. Soon the parents of those children were also covered. Middle-income residents earning less than $40,000 and those temporarily out of work were also included.

MinnesotaCare provided insurance to approximately 144,000 residents in 2002. A program that was projected to cost $1.3 million annually actually cost $390 million. Minnesota taxpayers financed 55 percent of the cost, primarily from a 2 percent provider tax and a 1 percent premium tax. The remainder of the financing comes from enrollee premiums, copayments, and federal funding. In addition, the young and healthy have seen their premiums rise by as much as 93 percent since 1992. Their premiums have increased $600 million to provide access to the previously uninsured.

Starting in 1996, the state commissioner was given the authority to institute price controls to hold costs down, and doctors and hospitals were forbidden to let per-patient revenues rise by more than 5.3 percent annually. Practitioners are strongly encouraged to follow medical practice guidelines in treating their patients. Such a plan was not feasible in 1987 when the legislative process began, but a carefully orchestrated system of reforms can get you where you want to go if you are patient enough. Once on the path of universal coverage, it is difficult to politically turn back (Henderson, 2002).

Hawaii's Universal Coverage

Hawaii legislated a mandatory employer-based insurance system almost 30 years ago. Under the Prepaid Health Care Act of 1974, employers are required to provide generous benefits packages for all employees working over 20 hours per week, but dependent coverage is not mandated. The employer must adopt one of two model plans or get state approval of an alternative plan. One option is the standard fee-for-service insurance plan offered by the states' Blue Cross/Blue Shield organization. The other is a health maintenance organization plan offered by the Kaiser Foundation Health Plan, Inc.

In 1991, the State Health Insurance Program extended coverage to those still uninsured under the Prepaid Health Care Act. Technically, these two laws extended coverage to the entire population. Because many Hawaiians hold several part-time jobs with different employers, over 11 percent of the state's nonelderly population is without insurance. Employers are required to pay at least half of the premiums and the employees are not to pay more than 1.5 percent of gross income directly toward the premiums. In addition, employers do not have the option of increasing deductibles or coinsurance because this would result in coverage that falls below the minimum standards.

A major complaint of the Hawaii plan is its inflexibility. In practice, all mandatory benefits must be provided, so any "optional" benefits are considered to be "additional" benefits. The Hawaiian economy is dominated by small businesses with over 99 percent of its employers having fewer than 100 employees. Due to a relatively tight labor market, many employers have found it necessary to hire seniors who would prefer to have long term care coverage rather than benefits for a younger population, but getting affordable options approved by the state regulators has been difficult.

Hawaii's situation may be unique due to the population's immobility and geographic isolation. Proximity to the Asian markets makes it attractive to business, despite the high insurance costs. However, administrative costs are lower because 80 percent of the population is covered by one of the two plans noted.

Critics of the Hawaiian system point out that total healthcare spending has grown faster in Hawaii than in the United States as a whole. Additionally, per capita spending is higher in Hawaii than in the rest of the country due primarily to higher Medicaid spending. Despite these concerns, the insurance premiums in Hawaii are among the lowest in the country. Further, annual cost increases among the predominantly community-rated plans have slowed to less than 10 percent.

Responding to the growing costs, the state legislation passed Health QUEST in 1994, which extends managed care to all public insurance beneficiaries and combines SHIP (Supplemental Health Insurance Program) and Medicaid recipients into a large insurance pool (Henderson, 2002).

Other State Reforms

Most of the other attempts at reform have not been as extensive as Hawaii or Oregon. Two-thirds of the states have enacted legislation to authorize small business purchasing pools. The insurance pools will provide small companies the leverage to negotiate more favorable premiums.

Several states, including Maryland, Montana, Vermont, and Washington, have taken steps to control expenditures on medical care by enacting limits on overall spending and limiting fees charged by practitioners. Legislation passed in

Maryland requires all insurance firms to provide a standard benefits package, with premiums based on community ratings, for firms of 2 to 50 employees. A commission has also been established to develop and implement a uniform payment system for all providers.

Clearly, states have taken the initiative in reform of the medical care system in this country. Many of the reforms, though, have been piecemeal and only try to improve access to the **traditional insurance system**. Given the lack of consensus at the national level concerning reform, indivisible states are viewing themselves as natural laboratories to test various reform alternatives. These experiments are important because they can give insights into what may be able to work at the national level.

UNITED STATES REFORM ALTERNATIVES

Three alternative strategies routinely compete for acceptance:

1. the all-government, single-payer option
2. **mandated insurance coverage** secured through place of employment
3. expanded use of **market incentives** to encourage and enable individuals to purchase insurance

Americans are almost equally split among these alternatives in terms of their preference. (Henderson, 2002)

Single-Payer National Health Insurance

Proponents of universal health insurance coverage prefer the single-payer national insurance program. Under this system, everyone would participate in a single plan, administered and financed by the government or some quasi-governmental entity. A basic benefits package covering all medically necessary services would be available to the entire public. This follows the Canadian model that strictly requires the ban on certain types of private insurance to put everyone into a single, equal, plan. The elimination of financial barriers to the highest standards of care prohibits any form of deductible or copayment. In contrast, the Swedish model allows private insurance and requires a modest copayment from patients when they receive medicals services.

Physicians would not bill patients directly. Instead they would bill the single payer account to a fee schedule determined through negotiations between representatives of the medical profession and the single payer. Hospitals reimbursement strategies vary considerably. Paid either on a fee-for-service or per-diem basis, hospitals are merely billing the appropriate government agency for reimbursement. If, however, hospitals are provided with global budgets, the traditional bill no longer exists. They become unnecessary because the hospitals get a periodic appropriation. The single payer establishes the budgets annually. Hospitals are required to treat all patients seeking care and spending is capped at a level established by the global operating budget. All capital acquisitions must be approved by the single payer and are typically paid out of a separate capital budget controlling overall investment in medical technology.

The theoretical model that applies to a single-payer approach is referred to as monopsony. Under a monopsonistic healthcare system, the government is the only purchaser of health care. This is not socialized medicine in its purest form because healthcare delivery is based in the private sector, but requires deep involvement by the government in setting global budgets for hospitals and nursing homes, establishing a ceiling on overall spending, and setting allowable fees for providers. Many proponents of such a system state that the growth of the health economy be limited to the overall growth of the economy, which is measured by the annual percent change of the GDP.

The main advantage of the single-payer system is its administrative simplicity. The only paper trail is between the governmental payer and the provider. In contrast, the American system is a myriad of payers and paper trails, making the system administratively inefficient. Another advantage of the single-payer system is that everyone is covered, regardless of financial or employment status, which again is in contrast with the employer-based system of the United States. Proponents argue that the single-payer system is the best way to strike a balance between access, cost, and quality issues.

Critics say that the government is already too involved in healthcare delivery and the single-payer system adds more power to the governmental side. A single-payer system results in a higher tax burden and because the direct effect of personal insurance premium changes are eliminated, individuals lose the responsibility to control expenditures. The benefits, as well as the expenditures, are spread over an entire system.

The argument for the single-payer system usually focuses on the duplication of services by a system populated by multiple insurers. The elimination of duplication will control costs due to greater administrative efficiency.

Employer-Based Health Insurance

More than 90 percent of the privately insured nonelderly population in the United States receives health insurance coverage through employment (Fronstein 2000). Therefore, many reformers rely on proposals that include the employer-based system.

Employer-Based Health Insurance

More than 90 percent of the privately insured nonelderly population receives health insurance coverage through the workplace (Fronstein, 2000). Given this tradition, many reform proposals rely on strategies that build on the employer-based system. The attractiveness of the employer-based system is based on three characteristics:

1. economies of scale are attained when administering to a large group
2. the workplace is an ideal place to pool risks because the workers are on average healthier than nonworkers
3. there is a favorable tax benefit for health insurance

Employers provide health insurance instead of increasing pay, which began during the wage and price controls put in place after World War II. The favorable tax treatment occurs because the benefits are not part of taxable income and are outside of the wage-price guidelines. This tax incentive put in place by the Internal Revenue Service (IRS) was upheld in a 1954 Supreme Court decision, and had a tremendous impact on workers' behaviors.

Employer-Mandated Insurance

Proponents of employer mandates have used this market-based principle to support their plan to provide universal insurance coverage to all working Americans and their dependents. One way of implementing an employer mandate is through the so-called "play or pay" approach. Under this scheme, employers would be required to purchase a basic healthcare package for their employees as defined by lawmakers. Employers would also have a second option. Instead of providing the benefit package, they could pay for a government-sponsored health plan through a new tax.

Even strong proponents of the "play or pay" approach recognize that equity issues arise because there is no mechanism for the unemployed. This approach would most likely increase the number of uninsured. In a study prepared for the Employment Policies Institute, it was estimated that such a mandate would lead to a loss of 3.1 million jobs (Bonilla, 1993). This mandated increase in labor costs would disproportionately affect low wage industries, such as restaurants, retail trade, construction, and agriculture.

Most firms in the United States already spend between 10 to 12 percent of payroll on medical costs. Public sector crowd out could occur if the tax rate for participation in the government-sponsored plan is set at a lower level than the current payroll expenses, in which case many firms would be motivated to join the public system of health insurance coverage. The Congressional Budget Office estimated that one-half of the U.S. population would ultimately move to the government plan, implying that the United States would have a system largely dominated by the federal government.

Individual Mandates

Instead of an employer mandate many reformers prefer an individual mandate. This is a legal requirement that individuals carry their own insurance protection, much the way that automobile liability insurance works for all registered vehicles. This mandate is preferred by some because it eliminates the free-rider problem (Reinhardt, 1992).

By taking the employer out of the business of supplying health insurance coverage, individuals would be more aware of the actual costs of their health insurance (Pauly, 1994). However, it is a myth that employers pay for health benefits. This cost is part of the cost of production and is passed onto the consumers in higher prices, seen in lower profits, or passed onto employees in the form of lower salaries or higher unemployment rates. In very competitive markets where the profit margins are very low, employees take on much of the burden of rising health insurance costs. Actual wages are lower and nonmedical benefits are less generous (Jensen and Morrissey, 1999).

Implementation of an individual mandate would require that employees who currently receive employer-paid health benefits would receive this portion of their benefits as gross income and then purchase insurance using these funds.

Market-Based Alternatives

Only the United States and the Republic of South Africa use the market mechanisms to any extent to address issues of cost and access in the health economy. Nearly all other countries have virtually dismissed the market as a means of delivering health care. Critics of the market approach argue that the market cannot be used to address a fundamental issue—the delivery of medical care.

The Market Approach

Advocates of the market approach do not see the growing number of uninsured and higher costs of health care as failures of the market mechanisms. Instead, they see it as a failure of the government to promote competitive market behavior as the cause of rising costs and decreased access to care.

The market approach is most closely associated with the tax code to make people more sensitive to the costs of medical care and health insurance reform, in order to improve access for the uninsured or uninsurable. Tax credits are suggested as one way to encourage low-income families to buy their own health insurance. This option would be limited to families with less than some percentage of the poverty income level, usually 150 to 200 percent. Critics argue that this is nothing more than a symbolic gesture and would have little real impact on the number of uninsured. Proponents do not expect miracles from their proposal, but think that the credit or even a voucher system would increase access for low-income Americans. The goal of market proponents is to improve access by establishing a mechanism that provides incentives at the margin to encourage some to take responsibility for their own care. In fact, many supporters of the market approach think that vouchers or tax credits could take the place of Medicaid or Medicare.

Many market proponents also think that the major distortion in the health insurance market is the tax treatment of employer-sponsored health insurance, which creates inefficiencies and inequities in the market. Because employer-sponsored health benefits are not treated as taxable incomes, employees are desensitized to the true cost of health insurance. The elimination of the tax exemption or some limit on the current subsidy would represent a major move in promoting public cost-conscious behaviors. In addition, this change could result in an increase in income tax revenues that could be used to reduce taxes, reduce the federal budget deficit, or finance other parts of the health reform plan.

A problem that limits insurance availability is that individuals and small businesses are fed into small pools for underwriting purposes. The inability to spread the risk into sufficiently large groups make premiums significantly higher because of the high costs of administering small risk pools, which are subject to large increases in the event of a single catastrophic loss. Another problem with current practices is that insurance is denied to certain vulnerable groups—job losers, job changers, and those with chronic medical conditions. Further, there is still limited access for the uninsured who have preexisting medical conditions. Insurance does not have to be affordable, even if it is portable under the Health Insurance Portability and Accountability Act (HIPAA) of 1997. States still make their own regulations regarding premium rate setting. A market solution to this problem must include measures to make it easier to form larger risk pools, concentrating purchasing power and spending less money. Specifically, antitrust laws that inhibit or prevent cooperative agreements must be repealed in order for larger pools to be established. Such changes would expedite the creation of **health insurance purchasing cooperatives** (HIPCs) to enhance access and lower the cost of insurance to individuals and small groups.

Another important cost control measure is the enrollment in managed care plans. Over the past decade, the private sector has increased its managed care enrollment to an unprece-dented level, but the same has not occurred for public sector programs such as Medicare. For example, less than 20 percent of Medicare beneficiaries who have a choice are in managed care plans.

The market-based approaches are built around the assumption that individual decisions are better than collective decisions. The market plan would provide more power to the individual, whereas the main alternative would give more power to the government. The real debate is between those who feel that individuals can be responsible for making medical care decisions and those who think the medical care system is too complex for individual decision making.

SUMMARY

Healthcare reform is a daunting challenge for U.S. policy makers. The people want change, but offer little consensus on how to achieve it. Government action seems to be inevitable, but the extent of the action is likely to fall far short of what anyone could have imagined shortly after the legislation was first introduced in 1993. It does not mean, however, that we have lost the opportunity to improve the system. This historic window of opportunity is not likely to close anytime soon. At least not as long as the public's desire for change remains strong.

However, it is unlikely that any comprehensive plan for government takeover of healthcare delivery will ever happen. Instead, there will probably be incremental reforms to add coverage and access to groups at the margin. For example, in 1997 Congress enacted the State Children's Health Insurance Program (SCHIP), which provides matching funds to states that provide health insurance to low-income children without insurance. Estimated to cover more than 2 million children nationwide, SCHIP represents the largest expansion of health insurance coverage for children since the enactment of Medicaid in 1965.

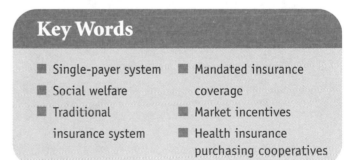

Key Words

- Single-payer system
- Social welfare
- Traditional insurance system
- Mandated insurance coverage
- Market incentives
- Health insurance purchasing cooperatives

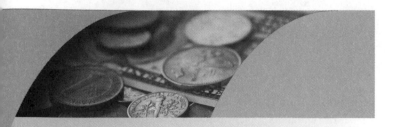

Questions

1. What are the respective roles of the federal and state governments in providing health services?

2. Is death an enemy that should be fought off at all costs or is it a condition of life that is to be accepted? How does the way we answer this question affect the kind of healthcare system that we might embrace?

3. In what sense do Americans have a right to medical care? In what sense is access to medical care not a right? How have reforms in Oregon and Hawaii helped define the right to medical care in this country?

REFERENCES

1. Blendon, RJ et al. (1995) Who has the best health care system? A second look. *Health Affairs*, 14(4):220–230.

2. Bonilla, C. (1993) The price of a health care mandate. *Wall Street Journal*, August 20:A10.

3. Donelan, K. (1999) The cost of health system change: public discontent in five nations. *Health Affairs*, 18(3):206–216.

4. Eddy, DM. (1991) What care is 'essential'? What services are 'basic'? *Journal of the American Medical Association*, 265(6):782, 786–788.

5. Fronstein, P. (2000) Job-based health benefits continue to rise while uninsured rate declines. EBRI Notes, 21(n).

6. Hadorn, DC. (1991) Setting health priorities in Oregon: cost-effectiveness meets the rule of reason. *Journal of the American Medical Association*, 265(17):2218–2225.

7. Henderson, JW. (2002) *Health Economics and Policy*, 2d ed. Mason, OH: South-Western.

8. Jensen, GA, and MA Morrisey. (1999) *Mandated Benefit Laws and Employer-Sponsored Health Insurance*. Washington, DC: Health Insurance Association of America.

9. Mahar, M. (1993) Memo to Hillary: Here's how to cure what ails our health-care system. *Barron's*, March 1:8–11.

10. Musgrave, GL. (1993) Emotions, politics and economics: an introduction to health care. *Business Economics*, 28:7–10.

11. Pauly, MV. (1994) Making a case for employer-enforced individual mandates. *Health Affairs*, 13(2):21–33.

12. Reinhardt, U. (1992) You pay when business bankrolls health care. *Wall Street Journal*, December 2:21–33.

13. Robinson, R. (2000) Managed care in the United States: a dilemma for evidence-based policy. *Health Economics*, 9(1):1–7.

BIO: ANTHONY J. CUYLER

Anthony J. Cuyler has spent his professional career applying economic theory to the study of social problems, particularly those associated with health care. He attended Exeter University and graduated with a major in economics in 1964. After spending a year at the University of California at Los Angeles as a graduate student, he returned to Exeter as a lecturer. Moving to the University of York in 1969, he is still on the faculty and is now Director of Health Development and professor and head of the Department of Economics and Related Studies.

In 1971, a steady stream of contributions began coming into the field of health economics. Nine journal articles appeared that year, which quickly established Cuyler as a leader in health economics in England and worldwide. Since that time, he has published more than 225 articles, books, and monographs, in some of the leading medical and economics journals around the world. Since becoming involved in academic administration, his research output has slowed, but he still remains productive.

In addition to a strong research agenda, Cuyler has played an important public policy role, most recently in the redesign of the entire system of public funding of research and development of Britain's National Health System. As a teacher and mentor, he has played a significant role in shaping the way a generation of British economists thinks about designing healthcare systems.

Source: Anthony J. Cuyler, curriculum vitae.
Health Economics and Policy, 2nd Edition. James W. Henderson. (Cincinnati, OH: South-western, 2002).

Public Policy and Health Economics

THE MARKET-BASED SYSTEM

The fundamental difference between the approach to the provision of health care in the United States and most other industrialized nations is that the United States is more market-oriented, and insurance coverage is less inclusive. When health insurance is offered to workers as part of their compensation package, it is a tradeoff for higher cash wages, and it is not a "right." In most states, employers are not required to offer health insurance to employees. Whether they do so, depends on the labor regulations between workers and employers. In other industrialized nations, people generally contribute to a system of social insurance, either through general income tax or payroll taxes. This is true in the United States only of the Medicare contribution, although personal income taxes also support Medicaid, the State Children's Health Insurance Program (SCHIP), the National Institutes of Health, and the healthcare infrastructure, including **subsidies** to hospitals and medical schools.

All societies ration scarce resources. Therefore, the question is what basis should be used to ration access to health care. A market-based system relies more heavily on the price mechanism as a rationing device. The U.S. healthcare system is a mixture of a market system and a system in which services are allocated on the other bases. For example, Medicaid and SCHIP do not use the price mechanism to allocate healthcare resources. Medicare relies less on it because services are so heavily subsidized.

Demand versus Need

The greater reliance in the United States on the market and **rationing** by price, rather than by the government, is paralleled by an approach in healthcare economics that focuses on supply and demand. Thomas Rice is critical of a demand-driven system (Rice, 1998). He questions the concept of consumer sovereignty in a situation where demand determines the direction of technology development in health care. These criticisms rely on the assumption that nonmarket-based methods can and should be used to prioritize and determine distribution of the resources that a society decides to devote to health care. This approach requires faith that there is a way of determining an objective standard of health needs and an appropriate distribution of care (Johnson-Lans, 2004).

Evaluating Efficiency versus Equity

Critics of a healthcare system usually evaluate it based on two criteria: efficiency and fairness (or **equity**). In most economic decisions, there is some degree of tradeoff between the two criteria (Okun, 1975). To use a previous example, pricing insurance using experience rating is more efficient than broad-based community rating because it relates the marginal cost of insuring the individual to the price of the insurance policy. However, risk sharing through community rating is thought to be more equitable because consumers are not penalized for poor health.

In the case of health care, equity and efficiency may also be complementary. It is widely believed that the social costs of health care for the uninsured are higher than if they were insured, given that our society does not generally refuse to provide health care to the sick, even if they cannot pay. It is argued that the uninsured do not receive health care until illnesses are more advanced and that this results in higher treatment costs than if they had access to preventive care or earlier treatment. Moreover, people without health insurance tend to overuse hospital emergency room services, which are more expensive than physician office visits for nonemergent cases (Johnson-Lans, 2004).

A good deal of research has provided estimates of the incremental costs associated with insuring the uninsured. A 1993 study by Long and Marquis provides an estimate of $28.6 billion (adjusted to 2001 dollars). Adjusting for increases in the number of uninsured between 1993 to 2001 raised the estimate to $35 billion (IOM, 2003). A more recent study by Miller et al. provides 2002 estimates ranging from $44.9 billion to $57.4 billion, assuming the spending of the currently uninsured mirrors that of the privately insured. If we assume that the healthcare utilization and spending are comparable to those of the Medicaid population, the range is from $35.1 to $38.1 billion (Miller et al., 2003). Both sets of estimates deduct the value of in-kind uncompensated care that this group would receive if uninsured.

The health status of the community also has public goods aspects because poor health is associated with lower labor force participation, poverty, and homelessness. Low health status is also associated with increased risks of spreading communicable diseases to other members of the community. The reduction in these indirect social costs that would be accomplished by insuring the uninsured should be subtracted from the increase in direct healthcare costs. A full cost analysis of the lack of access to health care also needs to take into account the losses due to shorter lives or a lower quality of remaining life years (QALYs) (Johnson-Lans, 2004).

The Rising Cost of Health Care

Increases in healthcare costs are an international problem. David Cutler pointed out that social insurance systems were originally more concerned with equity and provided most of what people wanted without a great deal of concern with efficiency. Today, this is no longer possible (Cutler, 2002). The common problem facing all industrialized nations is how to pay for the level of health care that their citizens want. Given the dramatic improvements in medical technology, people everywhere have rising expectations about what can be done to improve their health. The public healthcare systems are finding it necessary to cut back on coverage by limiting emergency care, and/or requiring higher copayments for services. With this trend, satisfaction surveys with health systems are much lower in most countries that a decade ago (Blendon et al., 2002; Donelan et al., 1999).

Technology Change and the Cost of Health Care

A number of economists have demonstrated that the largest contributor to rising healthcare costs are advances in technology. Although the cost of health care is worth it, it is important to develop strategies to identify particular components of healthcare expenditures that have low marginal benefits (Cutler and Richardson, 1999).

Technological change shifts the production function for health in favor of more health care versus other inputs. This has been the story of health care in the United States during much of the second half of the twentieth century. Therefore, there is no mystery as to why the total amount of medical spending is rising. A projection made in 2002 estimated that medical care would comprise 16.8 percent of the U.S. GDP by the year 2010 (Heffler et al., 2002).

The Role of Market Imperfections

The contribution of market imperfections to the cost of health care has been a constant concern in health economics. Critics have often associated a combination of **fee-for-service** payment and the lack of price competition with monopoly rents to providers. The healthcare market does not consist of small, perfectly competitive firms subject to long run zero profit competitive equilibrium. Instead, the markets for goods and services provided by physicians, hospitals, and pharmaceuticals are at best **monopolistically competitive**. However, price competition has increased greatly and was introduced largely because of the active role of third party payers, both private and public. Managed care has also provided a mechanism for negotiating fees with hospitals, physicians, and pharmaceutical manufacturers (Johnson-Lans, 2004).

Imperfect Information

Problems associated with imperfect information occur not only in the insurance markets, but also in the provision of health care. Integrated delivery systems may contribute to this because managed care subscribers often have little knowledge of the costs of the different services that they consume. One way to improve efficiency is for health plans to provide information about the costs of particular services. This is likely to be more helpful in decisions about **nonacute care** (Baker et al., 2003).

Another area of imperfect information that affects both costs and quality of care is the lack of systemization of medical records of patients. Also, there is the lack of formally-articulated instructions from patients about their desires for end-of-life treatment. A nontrivial proportion of the total expenditure of health care in the United States is devoted to keeping very sick and terminally ill people alive by artificial means that are frequently counter to their wishes, which can no longer be expressed. In many cases, the treatment is not regarded by the medical community, family members, or most members of society as humane (Johnson-Lans, 2004).

Inefficiency of Insurance Markets

Advocates of a single-payer system often point to the costs of administering an insurance system that consists of insurance contracts with such a confusing array of technicalities about coverage. A system of multiple insurers is administratively more expensive than a single-payer system. However, it provides more choice to consumers, as well as more problems of adverse selection. It is unclear whether streamlining and standardizing insurance coverage (which would require additional regulatory costs and limit consumers' options) would bring about a net improvement in social welfare.

A lower deductible on an insurance policy is inefficient when its marginal cost is greater than the marginal benefit of additional coverage. The load or loading fee is a much higher proportion of the insurance premium in low deductible policies. This is one of the reasons why some economists have advocated a combination of high deductible insurance policies (usually called catastrophic coverage) and personal **medical savings accounts** (Eichener et al., 1996; Jenson, 2000).

Experience rating is well-known form of achieving greater efficiency in insurance markets. **Price discrimination** is based on differences in the costs of insuring different individuals promotes efficiency in that it relates marginal costs and price. It is a common practice in the home owners', life insurance, and automobile insurance markets. Experience rating also removes the incentive to cream skim, the practice whereby insurance companies purposely select healthier clients (Johnson-Lans, 2004).

The argument for community rating is that risk sharing among members of the community is more equitable. It is thought to be unfair to charge people more for insurance because they experience unavoidable bouts of illness or deterioration of health. Because the purpose of insurance is to pool risks, experience rating, if carried to an extreme, undermines the goal of insurance.

There is considerable evidence that medical malpractice law in many states does not promote higher quality care, but contributes substantially to the costs of medical practice and encourages the practice of defensive medicine (Johnson-Lans, 2004).

RECOMMENDATIONS FOR IMPROVING THE EFFICIENCY OF THE U.S. HEALTHCARE SYSTEM

Critics maintain that there are few financial incentives for hospitals and integrated healthcare delivery systems to reorganize so as to reduce medical errors by monitoring overuse or misuse of medical treatments (Becher and Chassin, 2001). Drawing from the analogy using the U.S. auto industry, critics have suggested that the absence of competition of the kind that Toyota provided for the U.S. automakers has resulted in a lack of quality improvements in medicine (Coye, 2001). Physician groups within leading medical schools of public health, however, have been devoting considerable effort to designing ways of reorganizing clinical settings in order to provide more fail-safe checks on potential medical errors. Their point of view is that human error is inevitable. Failure to report such failures is due to fears of individual tort liability. If the system could provide checks so that errors could be detected before damage is done to patients, and if the institutions, not the individuals, were the focus of responsibility of medical errors, the organizations could be greatly improved to reduce medical errors (Weiner et al., 1997).

Information technology can be used in a variety of systems to improve the healthcare system's performance and efficiency. These include the compilation of patients' medical records, monitoring safety procedures in clinical settings, and dissemination of information to doctors about new technologies and biopharmaceutical products.

It is technically possible to have computerized records of patients' medical histories available online to patients, with password protection of the kind that is used for computerized financial information. Concerns about privacy and the reluctance of the medical profession to gear up to provide this kind of record keeping have so far prevented this system from being employed (Clinton, 2004). However, this would reduce unnecessary duplication in testing and reduce medical errors that result from providers undertaking treatment with lack of information about a patient's medication and general history (Johnson-Lans, 2004).

There are strong advocates of reporting systems that provide consumers with statistics on treatment outcomes. Some medical delivery systems, health associations, and government agencies have been established to perform this kind of monitoring. The Centers for Medicare and Medicaid Services are working on developing more programs in this area. Such programs may appear to have no downside, but critics of this innovation argue that it can lead to providers attempting to avoid treating the most difficult cases, or even falsifying records. Any system of reporting health outcomes of treatments must be carefully designed to adjust for severity of illness of the patient pool treated (Johnson-Lans, 2004).

A program that has served as a model is the Cardiac Surgery Reporting System in New York State. It has collected and published hospital and surgeon data on adjusted death rates following coronary artery bypass graft (CABG) surgery since 1989. It is operated by the New York State Health Department and is guided by an advisory committee. It has been effective in causing cardiac units to restrict operating privileges of surgeons whose patients have high mortality rates. Since this reporting system was instituted, New York has found to have the lowest risk-adjusted mortality rates following CABG surgery and the most rapid rate of decline in mortality rates following cardiac surgery (Becher and Chassin, 2001).

Many states have already engaged in legal reforms affecting medical malpractice law. Reforms that appear to have reduced the extent of the practice of defensive medicine include limiting the proportion of damage awards that attorneys can claim as fees, paying damages over the lifetime of the injured rather than in one lump sum, and establishing statewide pools to pay for serious medical errors even when they are not a result of negligence or incompetence (Johnson-Lans, 2004).

One reason why the healthcare spending in the United States is higher than in other countries is that on average Americans are less healthy. The proportion of low birthweight babies is much higher than in many comparable countries. The rate of obesity is higher. For the elderly, most of the healthcare expenditures are for cardiac disorders or cancers. Campaigns to improve health through better diet and more exercise could further reduce the incidence and prevalence of disease, and therefore reduce medical expenditures (Johnson-Lans, 2004).

Healthier lifestyles might also be encouraged by giving insurance discounts for healthy behavior. However, this form of price-discrimination is very difficult to implement in a system that is dominated by group insurance, where community rating is applied over the entire group.

Further, if it became routine practice for adults to establish healthcare powers of attorney combined with written instructions for the end-of-life treatment, this could reduce the per capita cost of health care, as well as provide utility to patients and their families. However, given the technological challenges in health science, it becomes increasingly difficult to specify what constitutes irreversible medical states.

The role of public health services is vitally important in controlling healthcare costs. The United States has failed to maintain vaccination programs for children at the level once achieved in the past. Both the private and public healthcare sectors have had much difficulty obtaining adequate flu vaccines over the past 4 years. Further, the emergence of multiple disease-resistant strains of communicable diseases, such as TB, requires a major public health effort. Prevention programs need to be in place, infected people need to be located, treated, and monitored. The research at the CDC needs to be maintained or expanded. The possibility of international crises, such as the severe acute respiratory syndrome (SARS) scare in 2002

and 2003, and threats of bioterrorism provide additional reasons for enhancing public health in the United States (Johnson-Lans, 2004).

Greater use of public health nurses and paramedical workers could raise the level of health in underserved communities and provide savings, by reducing the use of hospital emergency rooms. This is one lesson to be learned from the developing nations, where health workers are widely used to promote community health.

SUMMARY

The proportion of **GDP** devoted to health care in the United States and other high income countries is likely to continue to rise with improving medical technology, the shifting of the age distribution of the population, increases in longevity, and the fact that health care tends to be a superior good. However, if cost effectiveness is taken into consideration, the upward trend in healthcare costs is much less alarming. The increased efficiency in the delivery of care will dampen the effects of the increased consumption of services due to more incidence and prevalence of comorbidities.

Although there are many types of market failures in the production and consumption of health care, the rising costs of health care does not at present appear to be primarily the result of market failure. Those market failures that have occurred in the production and delivery of health care have been somewhat offset by the countervailing power of third party payers.

Technology, rather than market failure, appears to be the main cause of the increase in the cost of health care. Countries that have succeeded in controlling healthcare costs to a greater extent than the United States have done so largely through direct price controls and/or limiting the diffusion of technology. However, there are a number of inefficiencies in the system that could be overcome with the help of the high level of information technology available. Programs to improve the overall health status of the population could also reduce the proportion of GDP devoted to health care.

Key Words

- Equity
- Fee-for-service
- GDP
- Medical savings accounts
- Monopolistically competitive
- Nonacute care
- Price discrimination
- Rationing
- Subsidies

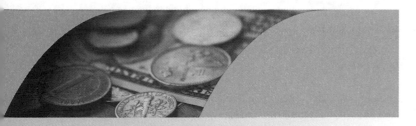

Questions

1. Approximately how much would it cost to insure the currently uninsured? Explain what costs are included and excluded in the estimates.

2. It has been said that employer-based insurance is obsolete. Give an argument for each side of the issue.

REFERENCES

1. Baker, L et al. (2003) The relationship between technology availability and health care spending. *Health Affairs*, (Web Exclusive, Project HOPE—The People-to-People Health Foundation, Inc.).

2. Becher, EC and MR Chassin. (2001) Improving the quality of health care: who will lead? *Health Affairs*, 20:164–179.

3. Blendon, RJ et al. (2002) Inequalities in health care: a five country survey. *Health Affairs*, 23:182–193.

4. Clinton, HR. (2004) Now can we talk about medical care? *New York Times Sunday Magazine*, April 18:26–31, 56.

5. Coye, MJ. (2001) No Toyotas in health care: why medical care has not evolved to most patients' needs. *Health Affairs*, 20:44–56.

6. Cutler, D. (2002) Equity, efficiency and market fundamentals: the dynamics of international medical care reforms. *Journal of Economic Literature*, XL:881–906.

7. Cutler, D and E Richardson. Your money and your life: the value of health and what affects it. In: Garber, AM, ed. *Frontiers of Health Policy Research*. Cambridge, MA: MIT Press; 1999.

8. Donelan, K et al. (1999) The cost of health system change: public discontent in five nations. *Health Affairs*, 18:206–216.

9. Eichener, MJ, McMillan, M, and DA Wise. Insurance or self insurance? Variation, persistence and individual health accounts. In: Wise, DA, ed. *Advances in the Economics of Aging*. Chicago: University of Chicago Press; 1996.

10. Heffler, S et al. (2002) Health spending projections for 2001–2011: the latest outlook. *Health Affairs*, 21:207–218.

11. Iom. (2003) *Patient Safety: Achieving a New Standard for Care*, November 20, 2003.

12. Jenson, GA. Making room for medical savings accounts in the U.S. health care system. In: *American Health Care: Government Market Process and the Public Interest*. New Brunswick, NJ: Transaction Press; 2000.

13. Johnson-Lans, S. (2004) *A Health Economics Primer*. Boston: Pearson Addison Wesley.

14. Miller, GE, Banthin, JS, and JF Moeller. (2003) *Covering the Uninsured: Estimates of the Impact on Total Health Expenditures, 2002*. Rockville, MD: Agency for Healthcare Research and Quality.

15. Okun, A. (1975) *Equity and Efficiency: The Big Tradeoff*. Washington, DC: Brookings Institution.

16. Rice, T. Can markets give us the health system we want? In: Peterson, MA, ed. *Healthy Markets: The New Competition in Health Care*. Durham, NC: Duke University Press; 1998.

17. Weiner, BJ et al. (1997) Promoting clinical involvement in hospital quality improvement efforts: the effects of top management, board and physician leadership, *Health Services Research*, 32:491–510.

BIO: JOHN C. GOODMAN

John C. Goodman received his PhD in economics from Columbia University in New York. His academic credentials include teaching and research positions at six colleges and universities including Columbia, Stanford, Dartmouth, and Southern Methodist. He is the author of seven books and numerous other articles on topics such as health care and social security in Great Britain, regulation in medical care, and economic issues in public policy.

Although Goodman's work can be deemed interesting and important as evidenced by numerous awards and honors, nothing could have prepared him for the notoriety he has gained in the application of one simple economic axiom:

People spend their own money more wisely than they spend other people's money. Goodman and a colleague at the National Center for Policy Analysis (NCPA) incorporated this idea into the financing framework now called medical savings accounts. Working with Phil Gramm and Dick Armey, both doctoral level economists, they crafted a Republican alternative to the Clinton reform plan that used the medical savings account as the cornerstone in reforming the way Americans finance health care.

In 1983, the NCPA was formed, but no one could have predicted that Goodman's research would place him at the center of a political firestorm that we call the healthcare reform debate.

Source: Chris Warden. "NCPA's John Goodman: Shaping Debate with His Small but Powerful Think Tank." *Investor's Business Daily* 10(95), August 24, 1993, 1–2.

Health Economics and Policy, 2nd Edition. James W. Henderson. (Cincinnati, OH: South-western, 2002).

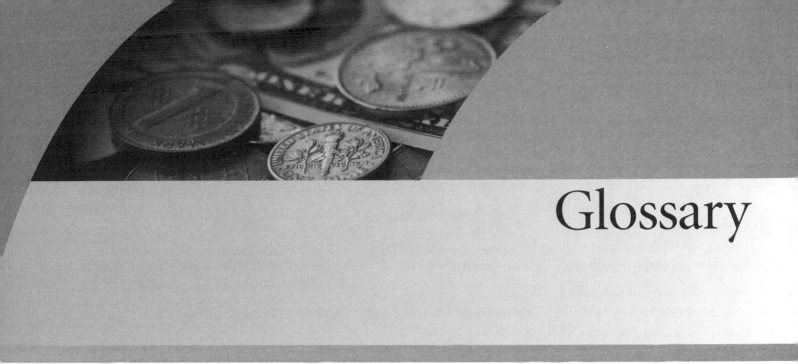

Glossary

Acquired immunodeficiency syndrome (AIDS): Results when the human immune system is so weakened by HIV that the body can no longer fight off serious infections.

Adverse selection: Exists when people with different health-related characteristics than the average person increase the amount of health insurance purchased.

American Medical Association (AMA): The major national association of physicians in the United States, whose mission is to promote the art and science of medicine and the improvement of public health. AMA was founded in 1847 at the Academy of Natural Sciences in Philadelphia. It is now the largest physician organization in the United States.

Average total costs (ATC): The ATC of production equals the total costs divided by the quantity of medical output.

Barrier to entry: An obstacle that prevents firms from costlessly entering a particular market. In the healthcare field, barriers can exist because of cost structure or legal restrictions.

Between-patent competition: May make changes in patent policy, such as the increase in patent life from 17 to 20 years, less important.

Coinsurance: A percentage to be paid by a health plan enrollee (beneficiary) of the cost of healthcare services.

Community rating: Applies when each member of an insurance pool pays the same premium per person or per family for the same coverage.

Comparative static: Examines how changes in market conditions influence the positions of the demand and supply curves and cause the equilibrium price and quantity to change.

Competition: Forces resource owners to use their resources to promote the highest possible satisfaction of society: consumers, producers, and investors. If the resource owners do this well, they are rewarded. If they are inefficient, they are penalized.

Cost function: A study that measures the total costs of a particular provision of services.

Cost-increasing technologies: Here, the increased use of medical technology can result in increased billings per physician.

Cost-utility analysis: Frequently used when comparing alternative drug therapies where benefits are measured not in dollar values but in units such as quality-adjusted life-years (QALYs).

Diminishing marginal returns: Additional units of investment are assumed to yield smaller marginal improvements in production.

Diminishing marginal utility: Additional units consumed are assumed to yield smaller marginal improvements in utility.

Diseconomies of scale (or Decreasing returns to scale): An increase in all inputs results in a less than proportionate increase in output. Diseconomies of scale result when the medical firm becomes too large and long run average costs increase, in other words when economies of scale are exhausted.

Efficiency: Measures how well resources are being used to promote social welfare.

Equilibrium: Demand and supply intersect with one another to establish market equilibrium.

Equity: Any right to an asset or property, held by a creditor, proprietor, or stockholder (shareholder).

Experience rating: This occurs when insurance companies base premiums on past levels of payouts, which is often done in the case of car or homeowners' insurance.

Externalities: Otherwise known as spillover effects, externalities are costs and benefits incurred in the consumption or production of goods and services that are not borne by the individual consumer or producer.

Fee-for-service: A method of paying physicians and other healthcare providers in which each service carries a fee.

Global budgets: A limit on total healthcare spending for a given unit of population, taking into account all sources of funds.

Gross Domestic Product (GDP): The market value of all goods and services produced by labor and property within the United States during a particular time period of time.

The Health Insurance Portability and Accountability Act (HIPAA) of 1996: An act making it illegal for insurers to exclude any employee from a group plan on the basis of health-related factors or past claims history.

Health insurance purchasing cooperatives (HIPCs): To enhance access and lower the cost of insurance to individuals and small groups.

Horizontal integration: A legal or contractual combination of buyers and suppliers, such as medical organizations, producing different medical services – for example different hospital groups.

Human capital: Equates the value of a human life to the discounted market value of the output produced by an individual over an expected period.

Increasing returns to scale: Results when an increase in all inputs results in a more than proportionate increase in output.

Indifference curve: Shows the various combinations of health and consumption goods that provide an individual with an equal amount of satisfaction or utility. A higher indifference curve represents a higher level of total utility.

Inferior good: If the percentage increase in the quantity consumed is less than the associated percentage increase in income.

Intellectual property rights: A collection of legal rights that may be used to protect an investment of creative effort.

Law of diminishing marginal product: An economic principle stating that as units of an input are used in production, a point is eventually reached at which output increases by continually smaller amount. In other words, the marginal product of the factor input begins to fall in value.

Long run average total cost (LATC): An envelope curve comprising the cost-minimizing points from a series of short run average cost curves. It represents the lowest costs of producing each unit of output in the long run.

Long run economies of scale: Refers to the notion that average costs fall as a medical firm gets physically larger, due to specialization of labor and capital.

Managed care: Any arrangement for health care in which someone is interposed between the patient and physician and has authority to place restraints on how and from whom the patient may obtain medical and health services, and what services are to be provided in a given situation.

Marginal analysis: Recognizes that choices are made at the margin, not on an all-or-nothing basis.

Marginal benefit (MB): The additional benefit received from consuming the next unit of the good or service.

Marginal cost (MC): The additional cost of consuming the next unit of a good or service.

Marginal efficiency of capital (MEC): A measure of how much extra output can be produced with an extra unit of input.

Marginal private benefit (MPB): The additional change in utility brought about by a one-unit change in consumption.

Marginal private cost (MPC): The additional change in total costs brought about by a one-unit change in factor input.

Marginal revenue (MR): The additional revenue generated from selling one more unit of a good or service.

Marginal revenue product: The marginal value or worth of an additional input, such as an employee, to a company. In a competitive marketplace, it is calculated by multiplying the price of the good or service by the marginal productivity of the input.

Marginal social benefit (MSB): The change in total social benefit brought about by a one-unit change in consumption of a good or service.

Marginal social cost (MSC): The change in total social costs resulting from a one-unit change in the production of a good or service.

Market: The characteristics of the buyers of health services; also can mean the geographical area to which services are to be provided.

Market failure: Arises when the free market fails to promote efficient use of resources by either producing more or less than the optimal level of output.

Market incentives: Inducement or supplemental reward that serves as a motivational device for a desired action or behavior.

Medical savings accounts: A mechanism created in 1996 by HIPAA to help individuals with a high-deductible health plan (HDHP) provide funds for health care.

Monopolistically competitive: A product market characterized by numerous sellers, moderate product differentiation, no barriers to entry, and some imperfections in consumer information.

Monopsony: A market in which there is only one buyer, and that buyer exerts a disproportionate influence on the market.

Moral hazard: Refers to the phenomenon of a person's behavior being affected by his or her insurance coverage.

New chemical entities (NCEs): Products developed by the pharmaceutical industry that historically have been based on chemistry rather than biology.

Normal good: A good for which income elasticity is positive but less than one. This means that if income increases by a given percentage, the quantity of the good consumed increases, but at a lower percentage than associated with the income increase.

Opportunity cost: The cost of any decision or choice made measured in terms of the value placed on the opportunity foregone.

Orphan drugs: Those used to treat rare diseases.

Output measurements: Conducted to make comparisons, either against other output measures or against some standard measure.

Pharmacy Benefit Management firms (PBMs): Act as intermediaries in the retail market for prescription drugs for insured patients.

Price elasticity of demand: A measure of the responsiveness of consumers to changes in the price of a good or service.

Price discrimination: Is based on differences in the costs of insuring different individuals promotes efficiency in that it relates marginal costs and price.

Private health insurance: Usually supplied by providers for profit, though it can also be offered by public bodies or by nonprofit organizations.

Production function: Identifies how various inputs can be combined and transformed into a final output.

Productive efficiency: Compacts the quantities of inputs used to produce a given output.

Quality-adjusted life-year (QALY): A measure used in economic and other analyses of the benefits of various healthcare procedures and programs, including drug therapies.

Rationing: A process of withholding goods and services when they are in short supply.

Risk-sharing: The division of financial risk among those furnishing the service.

Scarcity: Addresses the problem of limited resources and the need to make choices. Rationing is unavoidable, since not enough resources are available for everyone's needs.

Self-interest: The primary motivator of economic actors. People are motivated to pursue efficiently in the production and consumption decisions made.

Sexually transmitted diseases (STDs): A disease that may be transmitted by sexual contact.

Sickness funds: Which are private nonprofit companies, are responsible for collecting funds and reimbursing healthcare providers and hospitals.

Single payer system: A method of healthcare financing in which there is only one source of money for paying healthcare providers.

Social insurance: Workers, employers, and government all contribute to the financing of health care. Payments by employees can be fixed, or related to the size of their income, but not to their individual risk. Many countries finance their social insurance funds by means of a payroll tax, each firm paying an amount depending on the number of people they employ. The social insurance funds are usually independent of direct government control.

Superior good: If the percentage increase in the quantity consumed is greater than the associated percentage increase in income.

Supply and demand: Serve as the foundation of economic analysis. Pricing and output decisions are based on forces underlying these two economic concepts. Rationing using prices comes about when goods and services are allocated in the market based on the consumers' willingness to pay and the suppliers' willingness to provide at a given price.

Time preference: A term that refers to the extent to which people discount the future.

Traditional insurance system: A method of payment for medical services in which a medical care provider receives an individual payment for each medical service provided. This is a fee-for-service system.

Willingness to pay approach: Determines the value of a human life based on a person's willingness to pay for relatively small reductions in the chance of dying.

Within-patent competition: Occurs after patent expiration and also during on-patent time from firms in countries that do not enforce patent law.

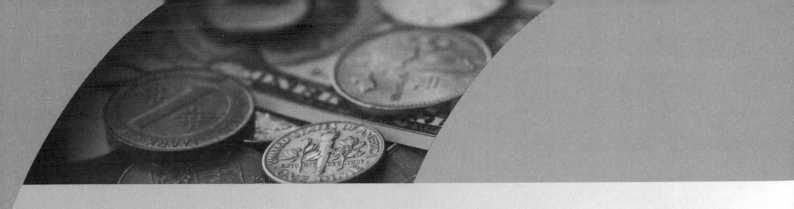

Index